Alternative The
Health Seri

I0016427

Juice Therapy

– in Everyday Life

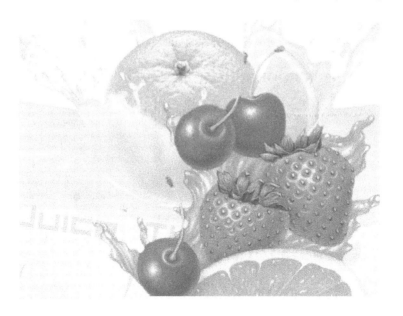

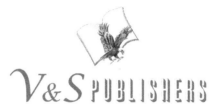

V&S PUBLISHERS

Published by

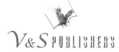

F-2/16, Ansari Road, Daryaganj, New Delhi-110002
☎ 011-23240026, 011-23240027 • *Fax* 011-23240028
Email info@vspublishers.com • *Website* www.vspublishers.com

Regional Office Hyderabad
5-1-707/1, Brij Bhawan (Beside Central Bank of India Lane)
Bank Street, Koti, Hyderabad - 500 095
☎ 040-24737290
E-mail vspublishershyd@gmail.com

Branch Office : Mumbai
Jaywant Industrial Estate, 1st Floor-108, Tardeo Road
Opposite Sobo Central, Mumbai - 400 034
☎ 022-23510736
E-mail: vspublishersmum@gmail.com

BUY OUR BOOKS FROM: AMAZON FLIPKART

© **Copyright** V&S PUBLISHERS
ISBN 978-93-579413-9-6
Edition 2020

Publisher's Note

Continuing with our 'Alternative Therapy Health series', we have now come to learn about Juice Therapy. "You are what you eat' – goes the proverbial maxim that forms the basis of phytotherapy or treatment with fruit and vegetable extracts. The modern nutrition gurus and dieticians call these extracts as 'nutriceuticals'- an umbrella term for dietary supplements. These are foods, as if especially created by nature for people with specific diseases. Besides providing alternative cures, these act as health tonics to supply vim, vigour and vitality.

The palliatives and potent curative aspects of plant products being natural in origin cause no side effects. Instead these products act as therapeutic or prophylactic medicines. Current researches by leading pharmaceutical R&D centres around the world have proved their indomitable power to cure or prevent large number of diseases viz., arthritis, high cholesterol, hypertension, osteoporosis, diabetes, asthma and more.

Kindly treat the below mentioned as a Disclaimer of sorts :

The Editorial Board writes in this book their opinion and that there may be many people who disagree with the conclusions. The publisher and the author, the distributors and bookstores, present this information for educational purposes only. This book is not making an attempt to prescribe any medical treatment; the knowledge given is just passing the acquired experience.

This book is only composed of opinions and conclusions of Editorial Board. The readers are requested to seek medical advice before blindly following the book. The Publisher/Authors shall not be liable for consequences therafter.

Preface

This book grew out to meet the burgeoning need for more professional knowledge about non-mainstream approaches in physical and mental well being. This need to spread awareness has been fueled by the huge consumer-driven trend toward these treatments over the last 2-3 decades. This text aims to provide a reader with cutting edge information from many diverse areas of alternative, complementary, and innovative clinical practice in the area of physical well being and emotional health. The purpose of this work is threefold:

1. To offer a broader, deeper view of information from areas that, although outside mainstream practice, are having an increasing impact and demand.

2. To offer a sense of the level of scientific research and experience associated with complementary and supplementary fields in the area of total health.

3. To further explore and incorporate new treatment options. This text, while not exhaustive, provides a fair overview from the cutting edge of change in health care practices. The overall layout of this 'Alternative Health Care Series' demonstrates the body-mind-spirit premise that permeates diverse field of treatment. By its very nature, this type of book is more focused on divisions and separations--different topics, different sections, and different treatments. Each section begins with a description of the treatment, its safety and/or contraindications, scientific documentation of its efficacy, discussion of which ailment it is best used for, and other important references. Time has come for physicians, clinicians and therapists to have a look at how the marriage of conventional health care to complementary and alternative therapies can offer improved diagnosis than either can alone. The text will offer them more knowledge, a broader viewpoint, and greater option to practice and care for those under their care and attention.

Table of Content's

ABC of Juice Therapy

Raw juice therapy in Naturopathy is a method of treatment of disease through an exclusive diet of juices of fruits and vegetables.

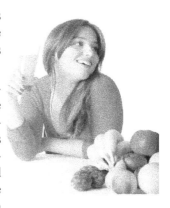

This therapy is considered the most effective way to restore health and revitalise the body. In raw juice therapy, the eliminative and cleansing capacity of the organs of elimination, namely lungs, liver, kidneys and the skin, is greatly increased and masses of accumulated metabolic waste and toxins are quickly removed. Digestion of food and the utilisation of nutrients are greatly improved in this therapy. An exclusive diet of raw juices of fruits and vegetables results in much faster recovery from diseases and more effective cleansing and regeneration of the tissues than the fasting on pure water.

Effects of Raw Juice Therapy

Raw juices of fruits and vegetables are very rich in vitamins, minerals, enzymes and natural sugars. They exercise advantageous effect in normalising all the body functions. They supply needed elements for the body's own healing activity and cell regeneration, thereby speeding the improvement. Alkaline elements in raw juice is highly beneficial in normalising acid-alkaline balance in the blood and tissues as there is over acidity in most conditions of ill-health. Calcium, potassium and silicon in raw juice help in restoring

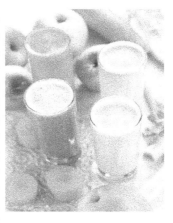

biochemical and mineral balance in the tissues and cells, thereby preventing premature ageing of cells and disease. Raw juices contain certain natural medicines, vegetal hormones and antibiotics. For instance, string beans are said to contain insulin-like substance.

Precautions in Raw Juice Therapy

Certain precautions are, however, necessary in adopting an exclusive diet of raw juices. All juices should be made fresh immediately before drinking. Canned and frozen juices should not be used. Only fresh ripe fruits and vegetables, preferably organically grown, should be used for extraction of juices. Raw juices oxidise rapidly and lose their medicinal value in storage, even under refrigeration so only 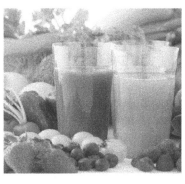 as much juice as needed for immediate consumption should be extracted. The quality of the juices has a distinct bearing on the results obtained. In case of incomplete extraction of juices, their effective power is proportionately reduced due to the absence of the vitamins and enzymes which are left behind in fibre and the pulp.

Types of Juices

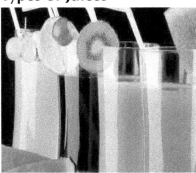 Fruit and vegetable juices may be divided into six main types. These are, Juices from sweet fruits such as prunes and grapes, Juices from sub-acid fruits like apple, plum, pear, peach, apricot and cherry, Juices from acid fruits like orange, lemon, grapefruit, strawberry and pineapple, Juices from vegetable fruits, namely, tomato and cucumber, Juices from green leafy vegetables like cabbage, celery, lettuce, spinach, parsley and watercress and Juices from root vegetables like beetroot, carrot, onion, potato and radish. Fruit juices stir up toxins and acids in the body, thereby stimulating the eliminative processes. Vegetable juices, on the other hand, soothe the jaded nerves and work in a much milder manner. They carry away toxic matter in a gentle way. Owing to their differing actions fruit and vegetable juices should not be used at the same time or mixed together. It is desirable to use juices individually.

Rules of Raw Juice Therapy

Raw juice therapy is a method of treatment of disease through an exclusive diet of juices of fruits and vegetables. It is also known as juice fasting. It is the most effective way to restore health and rejuvenate the body. An exclusive diet of raw juices of fruits and vegetables results in much faster recovery from diseases and more effective cleansing and regeneration of the tissues than the fasting on pure water.

As juices are extracted from plants and fruits, they process definite medicinal properties. Specific juices are beneficial in specific conditions. Besides specific medicinal virtues, raw fruit and vegetable juices have an extraordinary revitalizing and rejuvenating effect on all the organs, glands and functions of the body.

Who Should Avoid This Therapy

Juice fasts provide minimal calories and little fat or protein. They are not recommended during pregnancy or while breastfeeding, and they are also unwise for infants, young children, and the elderly. Certain health problems can make it necessary to avoid or limit intake of particular juices. For example, you should obviously avoid the juice of any fruit or vegetable to which you may have an allergy. If you have a problem with sugar, you'll need to dilute sugary juices such as carrot and beet with low-sugar juices such as celery. And if you have diabetes or suffer from hypoglycemia, you should always take fruit juices with food.

What Side Effects May Occur

Although, in general, there are no side effects from juice therapy, certain medical conditions such as diabetes may be aggravated by excessive intake of certain juices. It's also possible for a juice such as grapefruit to interact badly with certain prescription drugs such as Crixivan, Halcion, Lexxel, and Neoral. If you have chronic health problem or are currently undergoing treatment, it's wise to check with your doctor before undertaking juice therapy. Avoid including excessive amounts of tomato and citrus juices in your regimen. Because they are highly acidic, they could conceivably upset the body's natural acid-base (pH) balance. Remember, too, that the juice of a food to which you're allergic can be just as upsetting as the original source.

When Should Treatment Stop
Juice supplementation can last a lifetime. Juice fasts, however, should be limited to no more than 2 weeks at a time. No matter how many juices you include in the regimen, it will still lack many of the elements of a balanced diet. A protracted diet of juice alone will damage, rather than improve, your health.

Favourable Effects
The favourable effect of raw juices in the treatment of disease is attributed to the following facts. Raw juices of fruits and vegetables are extremely rich in vitamins, minerals, trace elements, enzymes and natural sugars. They exercise beneficial effect in normalizing all the body functions. They supply needed elements for the body's own healing activity and cell regeneration, thereby speeding the recovery.

1. The juices extracted from raw fruits and vegetables require no digestion and almost all their vital nutrients are assimilated directly in the bloodstream.
2. Raw juices are extremely rich in alkaline elements. This is highly beneficial in normalizing acid-alkaline balance in the blood and tissues as there is over-acidity in most conditions of ill-health.
3. Generous amounts of easily absorbed organic minerals in raw juices especially calcium, potassium and silicon help in restoring biochemical and mineral balance in the tissues and cells, thereby preventing premature ageing of cells and disease.
4. Raw juices contain certain natural medicines, vegetal hormones and antibiotics. For instance, string beans are said to contain insulin-like substance. Certain hormones needed by the pancreas to produce insulin are present in cucumber and onion juices. Fresh juices of garlic , onions, radish and tomatoes contain antibiotic substances.

Precautions
Certain precautions are, however, necessary in adopting an exclusive diet of raw juices:

1. All juices should be made fresh immediately before drinking. Canned and frozen juices should not be used.

2. Only fresh ripe fruits and vegetables, preferably organically grown, should be used for extraction of juices.
3. Only as much juice as needed for immediate consumption should be extracted. Raw juices oxidize rapidly and lose their medicinal value in storage, even under refrigeration.
4. The quality of the juices has a distinct bearing on the results obtained. In case of incomplete extraction of juices, their effective power is proportionately reduced due to the absence of the vitamins and enzymes which are left behind in fibre and the pulp.
5. If juices are too sweet they should be diluted in water on 50 : 50 basis or mixed with other less sweet juices. This is especially important in some specific conditions such as diabetes, hypoglycemia, arthritis and high blood pressure.

Fruit and vegetable juices may be divided into six main types.
1. Juices from sweet fruits such as prunes and grapes.
2. Juices from sub-acid fruits like apple, plum, pear, peach, apricot and cherry.
3. Juices from acid fruits like orange, lemon, grapefruit, strawberry and pineapple.
4. Juices from vegetable fruits, namely, tomato and cucumber.
5. Juices from green leafy vegetables like cabbage, celery, lettuce, spinach, parsley and watercress.
6. Juices from root vegetables like beetroot, carrot, onion, potato and radish.

Generally speaking, fruit juices stir up toxins and acids in the body, thereby stimulating the eliminative processes. Vegetable juices, on the other hand, soothe the jaded nerves and work in a much milder manner. They carry away toxic matter in a gentle way. Owing to their differing actions fruit and vegetable juices should not be used at the same time or mixed together. It is desirable to use juices individually. In any case not more than three juices should be used in any one mixture.

The following broad rules apply when using mixtures of juices:
Juices from sweet fruits may be combined with juices of sub-acid fruits, but not with those of acid fruits, vegetable fruits or vegetables.
1. Juices from sub-acid fruits may be combined with juices of sweet fruits, or acid fruits, but not with other juices.
2. Juices from acid fruits may be combined with those of sub-acid fruits or vegetable fruits, but not with other juices.

3. Juices from vegetable fruits may be combined with those of acid fruits or of green leafy vegetables, but not with other juices.
4. Juices from green leafy vegetables may be combined with those of vegetable fruits or of the root vegetable, but not with other juices.
5. Juices from root vegetables may be combined with those of green leafy vegetables, but not with other juices. A proper selection of juices in treating a particular ailment is very essential. Thus, for instance, juices of carrot, cucumber, cabbage and other vegetables are very valuable in asthma, arthritis and skin disease, but juices of orange and mosambi aggravate their symptoms by increasing the amount of mucus.

Method

When on a raw juice therapy, the prescribed juice should be drunk every three hours. One can thus take juices five to six times a day. A warm glass of water mixed with lemon juice, one teaspoon of honey, a dash of vinegar plus a small pinch of cayenne pepper may be taken first thing in the morning on arising to aid with the toxin cleanse.

Thereafter, the prescribed juice may be taken at three-hourly intervals. The quantity of juice on each occasion may be 250 ml on the first day. This quantity may be increased by 50 ml each succeeding day till one takes 600 ml on each occasion. The juice diet can be continued for 30 to 40 days without any ill-effects. The patient should take adequate rest during the raw juice therapy.

Raw juices act as a cleansing agent and start eliminating toxins and morbid matter from the system immediately. This often results in symptoms such as pain in the abdomen, diarrhea, loss of weight, headache, fever, weakness, sleeplessness and bad breath. These reactions, which are part of the cleansing process, should not be suppressed by the use of drugs. They will cease when the body is able to expel all toxins.

After the raw juice therapy, the return to normal balanced diet should be gradual, and in stages. In the beginning, two juice meals may be replaced by milk and fruits. Then gradually juice meals may be substituted by a balanced-diet.

Why Juice Therapy?

Fruits and vegetables provide one more substance that is absolutely essential for good health – water. More than 65% of most of the cells in the human body are made of water, and in some tissues, for example the brain, the cells can be made up of as much as 80% water. Water is absolutely essential for good health, yet most people don't consume enough water each day. Plus, many of the fluids we do drink, coffee, tea, soft drinks, alcoholic beverages and artificially flavoured drinks each contain substances that require extra water for your body to eliminate. Fruit and vegetable juices are free of these unneeded substances and are full of pure, clean water

Fruit and vegetable juices are good sources of the traditional nutrients. Citrus fruits (grapefruit, oranges, etc.) provide healthy portions of vitamin C. Carrot juice contains large quantities of vitamin A, in the form of beta carotene. A number of green juices are a good source of vitamin E. Fruit juices are a good source of essential minerals like iron, copper, potassium, sodium, iodine, and magnesium, which are bound by the plant in a form that is most easily assimilated during digestion.

Since juicing removes the indigestible fibre, these nutrients are available to the body in much larger quantities than if the piece of fruit or vegetable was eaten whole. For example, because many of the nutrients are trapped in the fibre, when you eat a raw carrot, you are only able to assimilate about 1% of the available beta carotene. When a carrot is juiced, removing the fibre, nearly 100% of the beta carotene can be assimilated.

Fresh juices are a tremendous source of enzymes. In fact, the "freshness" of juice is one of their key features, because enzymes are destroyed by heat. When you eat cooked foods, whether its meal, grains, fruits, or vegetables, if the food is cooked at temperatures above 114 degrees, the enzymes have been destroyed by the heat. Since fruits and vegetables are juiced raw, the enzymes are still viable when you drink the juice.

Restore Your Vitality & Revitalize Your Body

Juicing vegetables is one of the most powerful tools one can use to obtain high level vitality and the fastest way to restore your health. Vegetable juicing will establish an environment where nutrients can be used by the body. The nutrients are rich in supply and taken directly to the cells. Iron levels will normalize very quickly just on green juices alone. The benefits are enormous. The green juices in particular will build your blood, carry oxygen to the tissues and irrigate the system removing stagnation.

Live Enzymes & Living Juice

The simplest way to eat living food is drinking fresh juice. Fruits and vegetables build and regenerate our body; they provide minerals, enzymes, vitamins, carbohydrates, proteins, amino acids, and much more when eaten fresh or raw, without cooking or preservatives. Fresh juice is referred to as "live food" because it contains enzymes. Enzymes are protein molecules that have been found to have enormous health benefits. They have the ability to stimulate biochemical reaction. Enzymes are the body life force and are constantly breaking down substances and rejoining substances to rebuild and repair. Without enzymes all life would simply be a collection of lifeless chemicals. In other words, the element that enables the body to be nourished and live, the element that is hidden within seeds and plants in the sprouting and growth of plants, is a life principle known as enzymes. Heating enzymes and vitamins cause their destruction and minimize the vitality of your juice. Enzymes are the catalyst for the hundreds of thousands of chemical reactions that occur throughout the body; they are essential for the digestion and absorption of foods as well as for the production of cellular energy. Enzymes are essential for most of the building and rebuilding that goes on constantly in our bodies.

Fresh Fruit & Vegetable Juice for Your Daily Diet

The addition of fresh juices will immediately make our eating habits healthier by adding larger amounts of beneficial raw food in a delicious and more easily digestible form. Raw uncooked fruit and vegetables contain vitamins, minerals and enzymes. Dietary experts now emphasize the importance of vitamins and minerals for normal growth and tissue maintenance and efficient absorption (enzymes). The Super Angel is perfect for your diet depends on living and raw foods, especially hard-to-extract juices like wheatgrass and spinach as well as fibrous vegetables like beets.

The Benefits of Juice
♦ Improves life expectancy and health
♦ Contributes to the prevention of heart disease
♦ Helps with depression
♦ Helps relieve high blood pressure
♦ Helps detoxify the body therefore helps alleviate allergies
♦ Helps with degenerative and deficiency diseases
♦ Aids digestion
♦ It is believed that fresh juice may assist in reducing the body's stress by helping to correct acid/alkaline imbalances that are so common in our modern world.
♦ The nutrient and enzymes found in fresh juices can immediately go to work in the body to strengthen the body's natural immune system to help prevent disease.

Juicing Tips

More and more people are discovering fresh fruit and vegetable juices aren't just delicious. The advantage of drinking fresh fruit and vegetable juices is the health benefit of true freshness. None of the vital nutrients are lost when juice is consumed immediately after it is made. Just as important, no additives, preservatives, sugars, or sweeteners are added, and the juice has not been pasteurized to extend its shelf life. Fresh juice is absolutely pure, and you know exactly what it contains. The bounty of antioxidants in fresh fruits and vegetables, it has become increasingly apparent why it is important to enrich our diets with these nutrient-packed powerhouses. Today, this goal can be easily achieved with a few flavorful swallows, since drinking three 8-ounce glasses of juice can provide the nutritional benefits of up to 3 pounds of fresh fruits or vegetables.

Freshly juiced vegetables give your body an instant boost of nutrients, enzymes, vitamins and minerals in a form that the body can easily assimilate, absorb and digest – in fact, studies have shown that the nutrients from juiced vegetables are within our bloodstream within 30 minutes of consumption!

At the most basic level, juicing allows us to add so many more vegetables to our daily diet, and to up the amount of raw food we consume giving the body energy and boosting the immune system and the body's cleansing process.

Fresh juices are also believed to be a potent weapon against disease; studies show that juices can speed the healing of infections and can even help cure stomach ulcers. And when used in conjunction with other natural techniques, such as herbs, homeopathy and nutritional therapy, fresh juices can create an optimal nutritional foundation to bolster the body's innate healing abilities. High-Octane Nutrition. Fresh juices have more going for them than vitamins and minerals. A growing body of scientific research suggests that when it comes to the health benefits of fresh produce, vitamins and minerals may be just the tip of the iceberg.

Fresh Juicing Steps

1. Scrub produce thoroughly with a vegetable brush before juicing.
2. If a fruit or vegetable has been waxed, be sure to peel it before juicing.
3. Remove all seeds and pits. Make sure to peel citrus fruits.
4. Cut fruits and vegetables into small-enough pieces to fit easily through your juicer.
5. Wash and juice any stems or greens that are still attached to the fruit or vegetable.
6. Certain fruits, such as bananas and avocados, contain very little water and can't be juiced. Process in a blender instead, and then add to the juice.
7. For maximum benefit, serve juice immediately. Juices stored in the refrigerator lose their nutritional value quickly.

♦ Imported fruits and vegetables should be carefully handled because they contain more harmful pesticide residue than domestic produce.

Buying Fresh Fruits and Vegetables

At retail stores, purchase fresh fruits and vegetables that are not bruised or damaged. If buying fresh-cut ready-to-eat fruits and vegetables, be sure they are refrigerated or surrounded by ice. Fresh fruits and vegetables can become contaminated with harmful bacteria when they come into contact with unprocessed food items such as meats and their juices. Whether at home or at retail stores, be sure to separate fresh fruits and vegetables from unprocessed food items in order to avoid cross-contamination.

Washing Fruits and Vegetables & Preparation

Discard any rotten fruits and vegetables. Before and after handling fresh fruits and vegetables, always wash your hands thoroughly for at least 20 seconds with hot water and soap. Before eating, preparing or cutting fresh fruits and vegetables, thoroughly wash them under cold running water, unless otherwise specified – do not use soap or detergents; with a clean produce brush, scrub fresh fruits and vegetables that have firm surfaces, such as oranges, potatoes and carrots. Improperly washed fresh fruits and vegetables can become contaminated during cutting; cut away any damaged or bruised areas on fresh fruits and vegetables since harmful bacteria can thrive in these areas. Clean your knife after cutting these damaged or bruised areas.

All food equipment such as counter tops, cutting boards and utensils that come into contact with fresh produce should be thoroughly washed with hot water and soap. Rinse them and sanitize them with a mild bleach solution (5ml/1tsp. bleach per 750ml/3 cups water) and air-dry. Avoid using sponges because it is difficult to keep them free of bacteria. Immediately place peeled or cut fruits and vegetables on a separate clean plate. Avoid putting them back on the cutting board.

Pesticides are chemicals that are used to control pests that destroy crops. They are used in the production of most crops sold in the United States . These chemicals may increase your risk for cancer or other chronic diseases and should be limited in your diet. To reduce consumption of pesticides, follow these tips:

♦ Wash all fruits and vegetables with water
♦ Before eating apples, cucumbers, potatoes or other produce in which the outer skin or peeling is consumed, scrub with a brush
♦ Throw away the outer leaves of leafy vegetables, such as lettuce and cabbage
♦ Peel and cook when appropriate, although some nutrients and fibre may be lost when produce is peeled

Once your fruits and vegetables were ready for harvest, they were handled by several different pairs of hands in the fields and orchards, then in the warehouses and finally again in your grocery store. Listeria, Salmonella and E. Coli may all be lurking on your fruits and vegetables, whether they are organically grown or conventionally grown.

You need to get those fresh fruits and vegetables in your diet, but not the insects, chemicals and bacteria that come along with them so make sure you wash your fruits and vegetables before you eat them.

How to Wash Fruits and Vegetables
♦ Start by keeping your kitchen counter tops, refrigerator, cookware and cutlery clean.
♦ Always wash your hands before preparing meals and handling fruits and vegetables.
♦ Keep fresh greens, fruits and vegetables away from uncooked meats to avoid cross-contamination.
♦ Choose healthy looking, ripe fruits and vegetables when you shop. Avoid bruised, moldy and mushy produce.
♦ Wait until just before you eat or prepare your fruits and vegetables to wash them. Fruits and vegetables have natural coatings that

keep moisture inside and washing them will make them spoil sooner.

♦ Wash all pre-packaged fruits and vegetables, even if the label claims they are pre-washed.

♦ Wash all parts of your fruits and vegetables, even if you don't plan on eating the rind or peeling. Bacteria living on the outside of oranges, melons and squash can be transferred to the knives that cut them and then straight to the parts that you will be eating.

♦ Gently rub fruits and vegetables under running water. Don't use any soaps, detergents, bleaches or other toxic cleaning chemicals. These chemicals will leave a residue of their own on your produce.

♦ Commercial sprays and washes sold for cleaning vegetables really aren't any better than cleaning thoroughly with plain water, so don't waste your money on them.

♦ Firmer fruits and vegetables like apples and potatoes can be scrubbed with a vegetable brush while rinsing with clean water to remove dirt and residues.

♦ Remove and discard the outer leaves of lettuce and cabbage heads and thoroughly rinse the rest of the leaves.

♦ Rinse berries and other small fruits thoroughly and allow them to drain in a colander.

Remember that the fruits and vegetables you buy may look clean when you pick them out at the grocery store, but you can't see bacteria or chemicals. Your fruits and vegetables still need to be washed before you eat them or serve them to guests or family members. This is especially important for produce and greens that are eaten raw.

Storing Freshly Cut Fruits and Vegetables
Refrigerate fresh fruits and vegetables within two hours of peeling or cutting. Leftover cut fruits and vegetables should be discarded if left at room temperature for more than two hours. Prevent fruits and vegetables that have been peeled or cut from coming into direct contact with raw meat, poultry or fish.

Proper Storage Techniques for Fresh Produce
After returning from retail stores, promptly put away fresh fruits and vegetables that need refrigeration. The following are the different condition requirements for keeping fresh fruits and vegetables at their optimum freshness.

Only in the Refrigerator, Never at Room Temperature to Avoid Spoilage: apples, artichokes, asparagus, beans, beets, blueberries, broccoli, brussel sprouts, cabbage, Belgian endive, carrots, cauliflower, celery, cherries, sweet corn, cranberries, cucumbers, eggplant, ginger root, grapes, fresh herbs, leeks, lettuce and other greens, mushrooms, green onions, parsnips, peas, peppers, pineapple, new potatoes, radishes, raspberries, rhubarb, strawberries, squash, citrus fruit, turnips.

At Room Temperature until Ripe and then in the Refrigerator: apricots, avocados, kiwifruit, mangoes, melons, nectarines, papaya, peaches, pears, plums, tomatoes.

Only at Room Temperature and Preferably not in the Refrigerator: bananas, garlic, globe onions, mature potatoes, pumpkins, rutabagas, sweet potatoes.

Chapter 1

Acidity

Acidity refers to a set of symptoms caused by an imbalance between the acid secreting mechanism of the stomach and proximal intestine and the protective mechanisms that ensure their safety. The stomach normally secretes acid that is essential in the digestive process. This acid helps in breaking down the food during digestion. When there is excess production of acid by the gastric glands of the stomach, it results in the condition known as acidity. However, there are certain types of ulcers where acid secretion is either normal 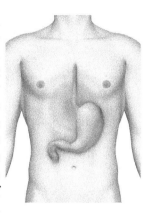 or even low. Acidity is responsible for symptoms like dyspepsia, heartburn and the formation of ulcers (erosion of the lining of the stomach or intestines). Acidity tends to have a much higher incidence in highly emotional and nervous individuals. It is also more common in the developed and industrialised nations, though a recent increase in incidence has also occurred in the developing countries. Consumption of Alcohol, highly spicy foodstuffs, non-vegetarian diets, and Non Steroidal Anti-Inflammatory Drugs (NSAID's) also predispose to gastric acidity.

Cause and Pathogenesis

The stomach, intestines, and digestive glands secrete hydrochloric acid and various enzymes, including pepsin that break down and digest food. The stomach must also be protected from the same acid and enzymes, or it too can be attacked by the gastric juices. The acid may enter the lower part of the Oesophagus (Gastro-Oesophageal Reflux), due to some weakness in the normal sphincter mechanism that prevents such reflux. This causes heartburn. It commonly occurs after meals and is brought on by excess intra-abdominal pressure like lifting weights or straining.

Ulcers also occur as a result of over secretion of acid. This may happen when there is an imbalance between the digestive juices used by the stomach to break down food and the various factors that protect the lining of the stomach and duodenum (the part of the small intestine that adjoins the stomach). A peptic ulcer is a raw area in the lining of the upper part of the small intestine (duodenal ulcer) or the stomach (gastric ulcer), whose protective mucosal lining has been eroded away by the gastric juices. Duodenal ulcers are three times more common than gastric ulcers. Hydrochloric acid, secreted in the stomach, is one of the factors in the development of ulcers, but is not solely responsible. Acid production in patients with duodenal ulcers tends to be higher than normal, while in those with stomach or gastric ulcers, it is usually normal or lower.

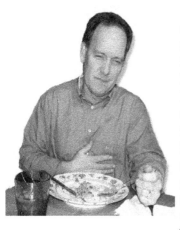

Excessively large amounts of acid secretion occur in certain situations, such as in a condition known as Zollinger-Ellison Syndrome, in which large amounts of secretion are stimulated by tumours located in the pancreas or duodenum. Pepsin is an enzyme that breaks down proteins. Pepsin and hydrochloric acid cause damage to the stomach or duodenum if the stomach's protective system is altered or damaged. The mucous layer, which coats the stomach and duodenum, forms the first line of defence against acid and pepsin. The body also secretes bicarbonate into the mucous layer, which neutralises the acid. The defence system also consists of hormone-like substances known as prostaglandins, which help to keep the blood vessels in the stomach dilated, ensuring adequate blood flow. Lack of adequate blood flow to the stomach contributes to ulcers. Prostaglandins are also believed to stimulate bicarbonate and mucous production, which help protect the stomach. If any of these defence mechanisms are deficient, acid and pepsin can attack the stomach lining causing an ulcer.

Symptoms and Signs

Dyspepsia and heartburn are often the main symptoms of acidity.

Heartburn is characterised by a deeply placed, burning pain in the chest behind the sternum (breast-bone). It occurs after meals and is brought on by excess intra-abdominal pressure like lifting weights or straining. It can also occur at night on lying down and is relieved when the individual sits up. The pain is very closely related to posture. Regurgitation of the gastric contents may also occur. The symptoms of ulcers are mainly pain that can be either localised or diffused. Sometimes it radiates to the back or to the chest.

The most common symptom is dyspepsia, a burning or aching pain in the upper abdomen sometimes described as a "stabbing feeling penetrating through the width of the gut". Rarely, there is no pain at all, but only a feeling of indigestion or nausea. Eating a meal usually relieves the pain in duodenal ulcer, but in a gastric ulcer there may be no change, or the pain may become worse. Peptic ulcer disease can sometimes occur without symptoms. Symptoms may also arise when there is no ulcer present, which is known as non-ulcer dyspepsia.

Investigations and Diagnosis

The clinical symptoms and history are very important aspects of diagnosis. Any present and past drug use, especially chronic use of NSAIDs, a history of family members with ulcers, alcohol consumption and smoking, stress assessment and analysis are very useful in determining the cause of the condition. A trial with acid-blocking medication is given with a four-week course of acid-suppressing drugs. In such cases, the symptoms may subside. If symptoms persist, then further testing is needed. Upper gastrointestinal Eendoscopy is done to detect the presence of ulcers. If Zollinger-Ellison Syndrome is suspected, blood levels of gastrin should be measured. Barium Meal studies are also useful as these may show inflammation, active ulcer craters, or deformities and scarring due to ulcers. If an ulcer is present, a precautionary biopsy of the ulcer is usually taken to rule out malignancy as it is not uncommon for a malignancy to manifest as an ulcer.

Treatment and Prognosis

Identifying and avoiding the causative factors are essential in the treatment of acidity. A suitable diet must be strictly followed avoiding spicy, salty and acidic foods. Smoking and alcohol consumption must be stopped. Those with highly nervous and emotional disposition and those involved in high-stress jobs must be encouraged to take lifestyle modifying measures. Antacids provide immediate relief of symptoms by neutralising the excess acid secreted. A group of drugs called H2 Receptor Blockers cause the stomach to produce less acid by blocking histamine receptors (example: drugs like Cimetidine, Ranitidine, Famotidine or Nizatidine). Another group of drugs called the Proton Pump Inhibitors, which selectively disable a mechanism in acid-making cells thus stopping acid production are more powerful and include Omeprazole and Lansoprazole. If ulcers have developed, they must be diagnosed rapidly and treated to prevent complications like perforations. Long term therapy lasting for weeks may be required to produce complete healing. Surgical methods of reducing the acid secretion like vagotomy are being used with decreasing frequency.

Prevention

Prevention mainly consists of avoiding the known causative factors like alcohol consumption, spicy foods, drugs like NSAID's, steroids etc. Patients with highly nervous and emotional disposition and those involved in high-stress jobs must be given psychological treatment. Avoiding non-vegetarian diets is also useful in minimising symptoms of acidity.

Beneficial Juices in Acidity: Grapes, orange, mosambi, carrot and spinach.

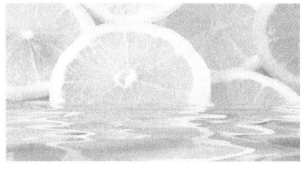

Effective home remedy for acidity using Lemon juice: You can take lemon juice in water several times in a day. To improve the taste, you can mix honey; do not add salt to it. If you are suffering from hyperacidity, do not eat food for 2-4 days. Take only the juice of such items as lemon, orange, mausambi, pineapple, carrots, pumpkin, cucumber, bottle gourd, etc. Lemon juice cures acidosis.

Chapter 2

Acne

A cne is a common chronic skin disease caused by bacteria. It is an inflammatory condition of the sebaceous glands and hair follicles usually found on the face, the neck, chest and shoulders.

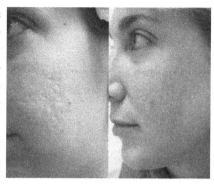

Acne is a skin disease caused by bacteria, which flourish on greasy scales. Nearly eight out of ten young people between the ages of twelve and twenty four suffer from some degree of acne. It is closely related to the disorder in the hormones experienced at puberty. Acne is an inflammatory condition of the sebaceous glands and hair follicles usually found on the face, the neck, chest and shoulders. The majority of patients recover between the ages twenty and thirty years. But it is still common in men over thirty years. In women, it rarely lasts beyond the early thirties and is normally worse before each menstrual period. All skin diseases, including acne, are the outcome of malfunctioning of the body as a whole.

Symptoms of Acne

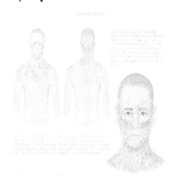

Acne is characterised by the eruption of blackheads, pimples, small superficial sebaceous cysts and scars mostly on the face. There are over half a dozen forms of acne, which are concerned with sebaceous glands or the glands connected with hair follicles. The most common form of acne is a blackhead, which chiefly affects the forehead, temples, cheeks, chin, chest and the back area. In rare cases, almost the entire body may be covered with blackheads with extensive scarring.

Causes of Acne

All forms of acne have their origin in wrong food habits, such as irregular hours of eating, improper food, excesses of starches and sugar, excess of fatty foods. Chronic constipation is another major cause of acne.

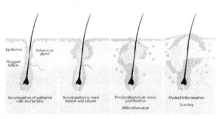

The extra efforts of the skin to eliminate excess waste result in acne and other forms of skin diseases. Yet another important cause of acne is a devitalised condition of the skin resulting from unhealthy living habits. There is also a general affinity among young persons to break and squeeze out the eruptions, which can only worsen the condition and help the infection to spread. Other causes of the disorder are excessive use of tea, coffee, alcohol or tobacco, strenuous studies, masturbation and sedentary habits, which lead to indigestion and general weakness.

Natural Remedy for Acne

In natural remedy for acne, the main emphasis is on diet and certain water applications. To begin with, the patient should resort to an all-fruit diet for about a week which should consists of fresh juicy fruits, such as apples, pears, grapes, grapefruit, pineapple and peaches. During this period, warm-water enema should be taken daily to cleanse the bowels and all other measures adopted to eradicate constipation. For complete recovery strict attention should be paid to the diet. Starchy, protein and fatty foods should be restricted. Acne can be treated successfully with two vitamins, namely, niacin and vitamin A. Zinc is another effective remedy in the realm of nutrition and it should be taken in therapeutic doses of 50 mg. three times a day. After noticeable improvement it can be gradually reduced.

Water Treatment for Acne

The patients should wash the face and other affected parts with plenty of hot water and soft soap to remove the excessive grease. Hot fomentation should be applied to open up the pores and squeeze out the waste matter and then it should be rinsed with cold water. A hot Epsom-salt bath twice a week will be highly beneficial in all cases of acne. This bath is prepared by adding one and half kg of Epsom-salt to 50 litres of water having a temperature of about 100 F. The patient should remain in the bath for twenty five to thirty five minutes till he perspires freely and after the bath; the patient should cool off gradually.

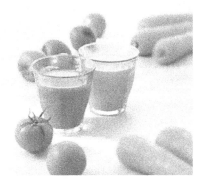

Beneficial Juices in Acne: Grapes, pear, plum, tomato, cucumber, carrot, potato and spinach.

Chapter 3

Anemia

Anemia is a decrease in number of red blood cells (RBCs) or less than the normal quantity of hemoglobin in the blood. However, it can include decreased oxygen-binding ability of each hemoglobin molecule due to deformity or lack in numerical development as in some other types of hemoglobin deficiency.

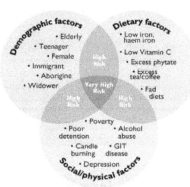

Because hemoglobin (found inside RBCs) normally carries oxygen from the lungs to the tissues, anemia leads to hypoxia (lack of oxygen) in organs. Since all human cells depend on oxygen for survival, varying degrees of anemia can have a wide range of clinical consequences.

Anemia is the most common disorder of the blood. The several kinds of anemia are produced by a variety of underlying causes. It can be classified in a variety of ways, based on the morphology of RBCs, underlying etiologic mechanisms, and discernible clinical spectra, to mention a few. The three main classes include excessive blood loss (acutely such as a hemorrhage or chronically through low-volume loss), excessive blood cell destruction (hemolysis) or deficient red blood cell production (ineffective hematopoiesis).

Of the two major approaches to diagnosis, the "kinetic" approach involves evaluating production, destruction and loss, and the "morphologic" approach groups anemia by red blood cell size. The morphologic approach uses a quickly available and low-cost lab test as its starting point (the MCV). On the other hand, focusing early on the question of production may allow the clinician to expose cases more rapidly where multiple causes of anemia coexist.

Signs and Symptoms

Anemia goes undetermined in many people, and symptoms can be minor or vague. The signs and symptoms can be related to the anemia itself, or the underlying cause.

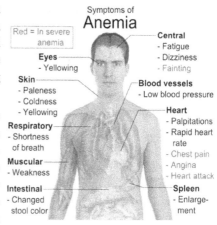

Symptoms of
Anemia

Red = In severe anemia

Eyes
- Yellowing

Skin
- Paleness
- Coldness
- Yellowing

Respiratory
- Shortness of breath

Muscular
- Weakness

Intestinal
- Changed stool color

Central
- Fatigue
- Dizziness
- Fainting

Blood vessels
- Low blood pressure

Heart
- Palpitations
- Rapid heart rate
- Chest pain
- Angina
- Heart attack

Spleen
- Enlargement

Most commonly, people with anemia report nonspecific symptoms of a feeling of weakness, or fatigue, general malaise and sometimes poor concentration. They may also report dyspnea (shortness of breath) on exertion. In very severe anemia, the body may compensate for the lack of oxygen-carrying capability of the blood by increasing cardiac output. The patient may have symptoms related to this, such as palpitations, angina (if pre-existing heart disease is present), intermittent claudication of the legs, and symptoms of heart failure.

On examination, the signs exhibited may include pallor (pale skin, mucosal linings and nail beds), but this is not a reliable sign. There may be signs of specific causes of anemia, e.g., koilonychia (in iron deficiency), jaundice (when anemia results from abnormal break down of red blood cells — in hemolytic anemia), bone deformities (found in thalassemia major) or leg ulcers (seen in sickle-cell disease).

In severe anemia, there may be signs of a hyperdynamic circulation: tachycardia (a fast heart rate), bounding pulse, flow murmurs, and cardiac ventricular hypertrophy (enlargement). There may be signs of heart failure.

Pica, the consumption of non-food items such as soil, paper, wax, grass, ice, and hair, may be a symptom of iron deficiency, although it occurs often in those who have normal levels of hemoglobin.

Chronic anemia may result in behavioural disturbances in children as a direct result of impaired neurological development in infants, and reduced scholastic performance in children of school age. Restless legs syndrome is more common in those with iron-deficiency anemia.

Diagnosis

Anemia is typically diagnosed on a complete blood count. Apart from reporting the number of red blood cells and the hemoglobin level, the automatic counters also measure the size of the red blood cells by flow cytometry, which is an important tool in distinguishing between the causes of anemia. Examination of a stained blood smear using a microscope can also be helpful, and is sometimes a necessity in regions of the world where automated analysis is less accessible.

In modern counters, four parametres (RBC count, hemoglobin concentration, MCV and RDW) are measured, allowing others (hematocrit, MCH and MCHC) to be calculated, and compared to values adjusted for age and sex. Some counters estimate hematocrit from direct measurements.

Reticulocyte counts, and the "kinetic" approach to anemia, have become more common than in the past in the large medical centres of the United States and some other wealthy nations, in part because some automatic counters now have the capacity to include reticulocyte counts. A reticulocyte count is a quantitative measure of the bone marrow's production of new red blood cells. The reticulocyte production index is a calculation of the ratio between the level of anemia and the extent to which the reticulocyte count has risen in response. If the degree of anemia is significant, even a "normal" reticulocyte count actually may reflect an inadequate response.

If an automated count is not available, a reticulocyte count can be done manually following special staining of the blood film. In manual examination, activity of the bone marrow can also be gauged qualitatively by subtle changes in the numbers and the morphology of young RBCs by examination under a microscope. Newly formed RBCs are usually slightly larger than older RBCs and show polychromasia. Even where the source of blood loss is obvious, evaluation of erythropoiesis can help assess whether the bone marrow will be able to compensate for the loss, and at what rate.

When the cause is not obvious, clinicians use other tests: ESR, ferritin, serum iron, transferrin, RBC folate level, serum vitamin B12, hemoglobin electrophoresis, renal function tests (e.g. serum creatinine).

When the diagnosis remains difficult, a bone marrow examination allows direct examination of the precursors to red cells.

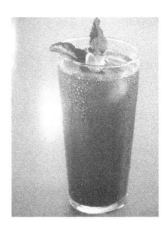

Beneficial Juices in Anemia: Apricot, prune, strawberry, red grape, beet, celery, carrot and spinach.

Beetroot juice, made from raw beets, is an especially good addition to any green drink. Beetroot juice contains phosphorus, sodium, magnesium, calcium, iron, and potassium, as well as vitamins A and C, niacin, folic acid, and biotin. When these nutrients are captured in a juicing process, they remain in a form that is much easier to assimilate than synthetic nutrients. For many years in Europe, beetroot has been used as a treatment for cancer. Specific anti-carcinogens are bound to the red colouring compounds, which supposedly help to fight against cancer. As far as the anemic is concerned, beetroot increases the uptake of oxygen by as much as 400 percent.

Chapter 4
Arthritis

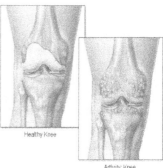

Healthy Knee

Arthritic Knee

A rthritis is a disease that involves a group of conditions in damaging the joints of the body.

Arthritis is a degenerative disease of the joints and a joint disorder featuring inflammation. This disease is common in elderly and obese people. Though, it is mainly the disease of mature age but nowadays it also affects the younger people. Arthritis is painful inflammation of joints affecting large weight bearing joints like knees, hips and also spine. The disease induces joint stiffness, pain, swelling and limitation of motion. Pain increases with motion and decreases with rest.

If analysed properly, many reasons will appear behind this disease depending on the form of arthritis. The reasons behind the disease include injury (leading to osteoarthritis), metabolic abnormalities (such as gout and pseudogout), hereditary factors, infections, and unclear reasons (such as rheumatoid arthritis and systemic lupus erythematosus). This disease is common to the people whose body's accumulation of morbid matter is of acidic nature. Due to the alkaline nature of bones, acidic morbid matter has a tendency to move towards the bones so that it could be neutralized by their alkalinity. In this process, it usually gets deposited in the joints and the symptoms of swelling and pain begin. In accordance with Yoga and Naturopathy, this disease may be the result of wrong eating, living and thinking habits.

The arthritic disease has a history that dates back to the ancient period. The mention of this disease has occupied pages in Atharva Veda and Charaka Samhitas. According to a great scientist philosopher of ancient time, the disease involves organs like liver, spleen, heart,

lung, kidneys etc. According to his observation these pioneers were well conversant with the fact that blood circulating through circulatory channels served as a vehicle for the spread of toxic material in the entire body.

This disease has some symptoms that are hugely discussed since the antiquity. The symptoms that are considered as primary include contraction, stiffness of joints, aching pain in the bones and joints, garrulousness, hunch back, horripilation, spasticity of hands, back and head, limping and lameness, atrophy of the limbs and insomnia. The ancient scientists have mentioned some more symptoms of arthritis. In children the condition tends to develop suddenly, many joints being affected from the beginning the small joint soft the hands ad feet being as a rule affected first. Arthritis can be both of the infective variety as well as the chronic. In infective arthritis the patient feels ill and toxic with a swinging temperature and a furred tongue. Leucocytes are always evident, and a blood culture may confirm the presence of the septicemia.

Proper diagnosis of arthritis is needed for apposite treatment of this painful disease. If the symptoms of arthritis long for two weeks, it can lead to acute problem of arthritis. The diagnosis will be based on the pattern of symptoms, the distribution of the inflamed joints, and any blood and X-ray findings.

Treatment

The ancient scientists and researchers have been offering treatment for arthritis in India. Several treatments which have been offered for this disease encompass Naturopathic treatment, Yogic therapy and Ayurveda. Naturopathic treatment includes water treatment, dietary supplementation and changes in diet, Injections, Herbal Medicines and Magnetic Therapy. In Naturopathy gentle massage is done with red oil to relieve pain, prevent recurrence and

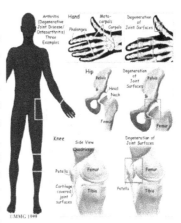

disability. This particular treatment implements well researched natural treatments such as diet, herbs, vitamins, and other holistic therapies that reduces the side effects of medications, reduce symptom severity and frequency. Treatments are different for the patients who are in the primary stage of arthritis and for the patients who suffer from acute cases of arthritis.

In arthritic treatment diet also plays a vital role. The practitioners of Naturopathy recommend a variety of supplements such as glucosamine sulphate and chondroitin sulphate, which are believed to rebuild the cartilage in joints. The diet intake should contain the recommended vitamins and on the other hand foods containing alkaloids should be avoided from diet as they interfere with joint repair and enhance inflammation.

Apart from dietary supplementation, the practitioners of Naturopathy treatment recommend injections of hyaluronic acid, prolozone, Traumeel, or Zeel into the affected joint. Many of these agents act to increase the amount of lubricating agent in the joint and decrease pain. The pain of arthritis can be relieved by Herbal Medicines suggested by the practitioners of Naturopathic treatment. The medicines that are recommended include natural anti-inflammatory drugs such as alfalfa, black cohosh, burdock, chaparral, Devil`s claw, juniper, and Yucca.

A much delayed but an effective way of the treatment of arthritis even of many disease is Homeopathy. The Naturopaths recommend homeopathic remedies that include bryonia, kali bichromicum, rhus toxicodendron, ruta graveolens, and ledum for treatment of arthritis.

Arthritis can be cured by the treatment of Yoga through practicing some Yogasanas.. Most of the exercises of Yogic Sukshma Vyayama are beneficial in this disease. Apart from the popular alternative processes the researchers of modern science have also discovered the ways to alleviate the difficulties faced by the patience till date.

Beneficial Juices in Arthritis: Sour cherries, pineapple, sour apple, lemon, grapefruit, cucumber, beet, carrot, lettuce and spinach.

Arthritis and Juice

Cherries have been receiving a lot of attention of late due to their beneficial effects on something that affects millions of people: arthritis. According to arthritis researchers, cherries contain anti-inflammatory properties that may work even better than over-the-counter drugs.

The Arthritis Foundation says that "drinking tart cherry juice mixed with water three times a day may be beneficial for some people with arthritis ... Cherries also contain varied antioxidants, including kaempferol and quercetin. These compounds, particularly quercetin, may have anti-inflammatory effects that are similar to those of nonsteroidal anti-inflammatory drugs (NSAIDs) such as aspirin and ibuprofen ..."

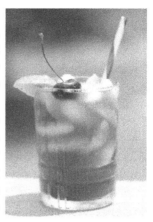

Researchers have focused their attention on tart cherry juice. According to a 1999 study by Michigan State University researchers, tart cherries contain something called anthocyanins that prevent free radical damage and inhibit cyclooxygenase enzymes better than some anti-inflammatory drugs that work as Cox inhibitors.

In order to inhibit Cox-2 enzymes, many anti-inflammatory drugs have to attack both Cox-1 and Cox-2 enzymes. Unfortunately, Cox-1 protects the lining of the stomach. This is why so many people who take anti-inflammatories on a regular basis develop stomach problems.

It turns out that cherries contain flavanoids and antioxidants that have a protective effect on the stomach, minimizing the deleterious effects of inhibiting Cox-1 enzymes.

While there haven't been any studies done on humans, researchers believe there's strong enough evidence to add cherries to your daily diet. They certainly won't hurt you and they might provide outstanding relief from the pain of arthritis.

Chapter 5

Allergies

Allergies, also known, as atopy is a disorder of the immune system that occurs due to allergens.

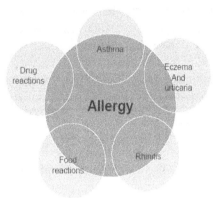

Allergy is basically a disorder of the immune system which happens due to allergens. Allergic reactions may occur within a few minutes of the patient coming in contact with the allergen, or they may be delayed for several hours or even several days.

Almost any part of the body can be affected by allergies, but the most common of them are the nose, the eyes, the skin, chest, intestines and ears. Allergies occur due to sensitiveness of the body to a substance, which does not normally affect other persons. There are innumerable substances in the environment, which can cause mild reactions, ranging from true allergies due to intolerance of certain foods and substances to violent reactions, in many people resulting from pollution.

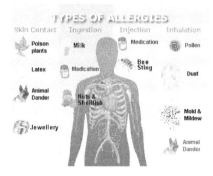

In ancient India, all forms of antipathy were classified as allergies, and all were caused by an improper activation of the immune system and natural herbs and minerals were believed to be the common treatment for allergies. Much later, it became clear that several different disease mechanisms were mixed up, with the common link to a disordered activation of the immune system. After many researchers in India since decades, allergy was described to be a hyperactive response of the immune system to certain substances, which are "foreign" to the human bodies. These substances are called "allergens", and they can range from food and pollen to dust and drugs.

After much research the symptom of allergy has been identified. The symptoms range at a great variety and vary according to the cause of allergy. These include recurring headache, migraine, dizziness, irritability, nervousness, depression, neuralgia, sneezing, conjunctivitis, diabetes, eczema, heart burn, hay fever, indigestion, constipation, diarrhoea, gastric ulcer, asthma, overweight, high blood pressure, chest pain, heart attacks, a stuffy or running nose, shortage of breath, swelling of the face and eyes, etc. The same food can cause different symptoms in different people. Many allergies are multiple and may be caused by multiple allergens.

A wide range of substances and conditions causes allergic reactions. These include pollen, dust, cosmetics and animal hair, poisonous plants, serums, vaccines and drugs, physical agents such as heat, cold and sunlight; as well as a variety of foods. Among the numerous allergens in edibles, the more common ones are oranges, milk, eggs, wheat, fish, chocolates, cabbage, potatoes, tomatoes and strawberries. Allergy is mostly caused by dietetic errors and faulty style of living. For instance, feeding babies are given artificial foodstuff like cereals, meat, corns, whole milk, etc. instead of mother's milk, before they reach the age of 10 to 12 months. Without proper enzymes needed for the digestion of such food at a very young age, these foods cause allergic reactions.

Another important cause of allergy is contemporary processed foods loaded with numerous chemical additives, many of which cause powerful reactions. An allergic condition can result from diet imbalances. There can be a breakdown in the body's ability to handle sugar due to excessive intake of refined sugar and consequent blood sugar irregularities, or mineral and vitamin imbalances due to defective dietary patterns. Emotional and psychological stress can also lead to allergies. A person through chronic stress can become sensitive to common foods or commonplace substances like petrol fumes.

The allergies are supposed to be tackled by every person. Hence, first the sources of the allergies must be identified, once the sources are discovered, they should be avoided and lastly, general health and resistance should be built up to establish immunity to them. People can also detect the disturbing foods, naturally, either by the trial-and-error elimination diet and a self-search method. This automatically eliminates many hazards and foods. One should keep away from the inorganic, untreated, unprocessed foods as far as possible.

The self-searched method is to be carried out to determine any suspicious symptoms from foods. It is advisable to try an eliminatory diet, excluding suspected foods for two weeks until the cause is detected. Occasionally, by changing the brand or the type, one can find a food substitute that does not upset the individual. The best way, however, to prevent or overcome allergies is to strengthen the overall physical resistance so as not to fall an easy prey to every allergen that comes along.

Diet can be one of the most favourable ways of avoiding allergies. The patient should fast on fresh fruit juices for four or five days. Repeated short juice fasts are likely to result in better tolerance to previous allergies. After the fruit juice fast for about a week the patient can take a mono diet of vegetables or fruits such as carrots, grapes or apples. After that one more food is added to the mono diet. A week later the third food is added and so on. After four weeks, the protein foods can be introduced, one at a time and in case an allergic reaction to a newly introduced food is noticed, it should be discontinued and a new food tried. In this way all real allergens can be eventually eliminated from the diet.

The foods which should be excluded from the diet are tea, coffee, chocolate, cola drinks, alcohol, sugar, sweets and foods containing sugar, refined cereals, meats, fish, chicken, tobacco, milk, cheese, butter, smoked, salted, pickled foods and foods containing any chemical additives, preservatives and flavouring. These foods cause either toxic accumulations or over-stimulation of adrenal glands or strain on pancreatic enzyme production or disturb the blood sugar balance.

For preventive purposes, the entire C complex vitamins are recommended. They gradually strengthen cell permeability to help immunize the body from various allergies, especially hay fever. Often the addition of pantothenic acid brings great relief to allergy sufferers. Multiple allergies may result from poor adrenal gland functioning. In such cases liberal amounts of pantothenic acids help cure them, although the recovery will take several weeks. An adequate intake of vitamin E is also beneficial, as this vitamin possesses effective anti-allergic properties.

The body requires a large alkaline reserve for its daily activity. The many emergencies of acid formation through the day from wrong foods; fatigue, mental stress and lack of sleep can be met by the competency of the alkaline reserves. Boosting the normal body reserve of alkaline by liberal use of alkaline-forming foods is essential for those suffering from allergies. Treatment of Allergies by Yogic Asanas is also very effective. For allergic conditions in which an element of stress is present, it is essential to employ such methods as relaxation, exercise, meditation and mind control. These methods will reduce or remove stress and thereby contribute towards the treatment of allergies. Yogic asanas like yogamudra ardh-matsyendrasana, sarvangasana, shavasana and anuloma- viloma, pranayama are also beneficial. Magnetic Therapy, being one of the treatment methods of allergies, suggests people suffering from allergy should take mixed magnetised water regularly. They should also apply the magnets twice daily for 15 minutes once to the hands in the morning and again to the thighs (about 5 cm above the upper border of the patella on the inner side) with North Pole placed on the right thigh and South Pole on the left. The recommended treatment is suitable for any type of allergy.

Allergies are a common trouble faced by most of the people in India due to various causes. With the advancement of medical science, many methods of treatment are introduced in the area of allergies.

Beneficial Juices in Allergies: Apricot, grapes, carrot, beet and spinach.

Allergies treatment using Vegetable Juices

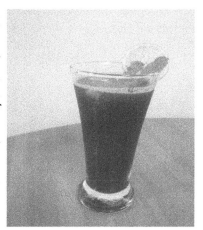

A quantity of 500 ml carrot juice or a combination of carrot juice with beet and cucumber juices, has been found beneficial in the treatment of allergies. In the case of mixed juices, 100 ml each of beet and cucumber juices should be mixed with 300 ml of carrot juice to prepare 500 ml or half a litre of mixed juice. This should be taken once daily.

Arteriosclerosis

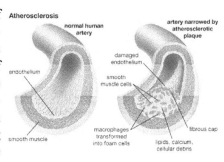

Atherosclerosis

normal human artery

artery narrowed by atherosclerotic plaque

damaged endothelium

endothelium

smooth muscle cells

smooth muscle

macrophages transformed into foam cells

lipids, calcium, cellular debris

fibrous cap

Arteriosclerosis is one of the most common diseases of the blood vessels. It refers to a thickening of the walls of the arteries due to the presence of calcium or lime. Arteriosclerosis is a kind of degeneration or softening of the inner lining of the blood vessel walls. The most risky places for such degeneration are the coronary vessels of the heart and the arteries leading to the brain.

It has been estimated that 40 per cent of all men over 40 years have a significant degree of obstruction of their coronary arteries and this can lead to heart attacks at any time. Arteriosclerosis results in the loss of elasticity of the blood vessels, with a narrowing of the smaller arteries, which interferes with the free circulation of the blood. These changes may gradually extend to capillaries and veins. Arteriosclerosis is more frequent in men than women, especially in the younger age group.

Symptoms of Arteriosclerosis

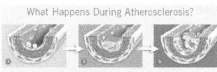

What Happens During Atherosclerosis?

Inflammation is a key factor in the development of atherosclerosis. ❶ As LDL cholesterol accumulates in the arterial wall, it undergoes chemical changes and signals to endothelial cells to latch onto white blood cells circulating in the blood. These immune cells penetrate the intima and trigger an inflammatory response, devouring LDLs, to become fat-laden "foam cells" and ❷ form a fatty streak, the earliest stage of atherosclerosis plaque. ❸ The plaque continues to grow and forms a fibrous cap. Substances released by foam cells can eventually destabilize the cap, allowing it to rupture, causing a blood clot which can block blood flow and trigger a heart attack.

The symptoms of arteriosclerosis vary with arteries involved. Signs of inadequate blood supply generally appear first in the legs. There may be numbness and coldness in the feet and cramps and pains in the legs even after light exercise. If the coronary arteries are involved, the patient may have sharp pains, characteristic of angina pectoris. When arteries leading to the brain are involved, the vessel may burst, causing haemorrhage in the brain tissues. A cerebral vascular stroke, with partial or complete paralysis of one side of the body may result, if there is blockage with a blood clot. It may also lead to loss of memory and a confused state of mind in elderly people. If arteries leading to the kidneys are involved, the patient may suffer from high blood pressure and kidney disorders.

Causes of Arteriosclerosis

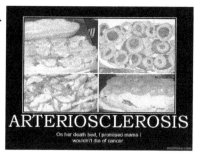

The most important cause of arteriosclerosis is excessive intake of white sugar, refined foods and high fat diet, rich in cholesterol. A sedentary life and excesses of all kinds are the major contributing causes. Other diseases such as high blood pressure, obesity, diabetes, rheumatism, malaria and syphilis may also cause hardening of the arteries. Emotional stress also plays an important part, and heart attacks are more common during the periods of mental and emotional disturbances, particularly in those engaged in sedentary occupations. Heredity also plays its role and this disease runs in families.

Treatment of Arteriosclerosis by Nature Cure:

Juice Diet:

The patient should resort to a short juice fast for five to seven days. All available fresh, raw vegetables and fruit juices in season may be taken. Grapefruit juice, pineapple juice, lemon juice and juices of green vegetables are especially beneficial. A warm water enema should be used daily to cleanse the bowels during the period of fasting. After the juice fast, the patient should take optimum diet made up from three basic food groups, namely (i) seeds, nuts and grains, (ii) vegetables and, (!!!) fruits, with emphasis on raw foods. Plenty of raw and sprouted seeds and nuts should be used. Cold pressed vegetable oils; particularly safflower oil, flax seed oil and olive oil should be used regularly.

Further, short fasts on juices may be undertaken at intervals of three months or so, depending on the progress being made. Instead of few large meals a patient should take frequent small meals. The patient should however, avoid all hydrogenated fats and an excess of saturated fats, such as butter, cream, ghee and animal fat. He should also avoid meat, salt and all refined and processed foods, condiments, sauces, pickles, strong tea, coffee, white sugar, white flour and all products made from them. Foods cooked in aluminum and copper utensils should not be taken, as toxic metals entering the body get deposited on the walls of the aorta and the arteries. Smoking, if habitual, should be given up as smoking constricts the arteries and aggravates the condition.

Beneficial Juices in Arteriosclerosis: Grapefruit, pineapple, lemon, celery, carrot, lettuce, and spinach.

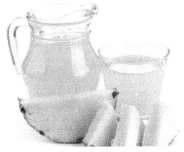

The beet juice has also proved valuable in arteriosclerosis. It is an excellent solvent for inorganic calcium deposits. Juices of carrot and spinach are also beneficial. These juices can be taken individually or in combination. Formula proportions found helpful when used in combination are 300 ml carrot and 200 ml spinach to prepare 500 ml of juice.

Chapter 7
Asthma

Asthma is a disease that affects the lungs and the airways that deliver air to the lungs. It causes periodic attacks of wheezing and difficult breathing. An asthma attack occurs when the airways become inflamed in response to a trigger, such as dust, mold, pets, exercise or cold weather. The latter may inflame the airways to the lungs, and the

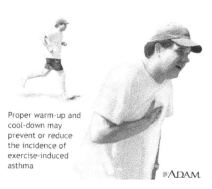

Proper warm-up and cool-down may prevent or reduce the incidence of exercise-induced asthma

mucous membrane covering the walls becomes swollen with fluid allowing disease-fighting cells to accumulate and causing swelling in the lungs. For this, the airways become blocked or obstructed when the muscles surrounding the lungs tighten or go into spasm. Due to the blockage, air cannot flow in and out of the lungs freely and a whistling or wheezing sound may be heard. Such attacks can be mild, moderate, or severe, and can last for a few minutes, a few hours, or several days.

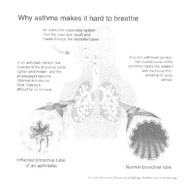

Why asthma makes it hard to breathe

Inflamed bronchial tube of an asthmatic

Normal bronchial tube

Some of the symptoms of Asthma include breathlessness at the time of attack, heaviness in the chest, distended abdomen, uneasiness in body and increase in palpitation, cold and cough, weakness, breathing trouble during sleep and feeling of some comfort during sitting. The main causes of Asthma are the digestive disorders. If the food is not digested properly, it produces toxic juices in the system and causes obstructions in the respiratory tract resulting in the state of breathlessness.

Sometimes due to persistent Common Cold and cough, the symptoms of Asthma appear. If the parents have been the patients of Asthma their children may also develop this disease. Sometimes the effect of climate or some other disorders can also become the cause of Asthma.

An acute aggravation of asthma is commonly referred to as an asthma attack. The clinical hallmarks of an attack are shortness of breath called the dyspnea and either wheezing or stridor. Although the former is "often regarded as the sine qua non of asthma", some patients present mainly with coughing, and in the late stages of an attack, air motion may be so impaired that no wheezing may be heard. The onset of asthma may be sudden, with a sense of constriction in the chest, breathing becomes difficult, and wheezing occurs. During a serious asthma attack, the accessory muscles of respiration may be used, shown as in drawing of tissues between the ribs and above the sternum and clavicles.

During very severe asthma attacks, an asthma sufferer can turn blue from lack of oxygen and can experience chest pain or even loss of consciousness. Just before loss of consciousness, there is a chance that the patient will start to feel numbness in the limbs and palms and may also start to sweat. The person's feet may become icy cold. Severe asthma attacks, which may not be responsive to standard treatments are life threatening and may lead to respiratory arrest and death. Despite the severity of symptoms during an asthmatic episode, between attacks an asthmatic may show few or even no signs of the disease.

In several cases, a physician can diagnose asthma depending on typical findings in a patient's clinical history and examination. Asthma is strongly suspected if a patient suffers from eczema or other allergic conditions, thus suggesting a general atopic constitution or has a family history of asthma. While measurement of airway function is possible for adults, most new cases are diagnosed in children who are unable to perform such tests. Diagnosis in children is based on a careful compilation and analysis of the patient's medical history and subsequent improvement with an inhaled bronchodilator medication. In case of adults, diagnosis can be made with a peak flow metre, which tests airway restriction, checking both the diurnal variation and any reversibility following inhaled bronchodilator medication.

Treatment of Asthma

Treatment of Asthma can be done by nature cure. The first option is usually diet. The patient of Asthma should find out the measures to cleanse the bowel and respiratory tract by fasting for about one to two days and gradually come to liquid and fruit, diet. Regular warm water enema may be taken daily during fast. Thereafter normal diet

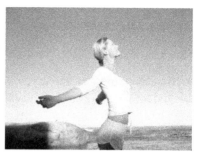

consisting of whole wheat bread and bottle gourd vegetable may be taken. Cold and heavy meal should be avoided and the dinner should be very light, honey can also be taken. Efforts should be made to have dinner before sunset. Warm water should be used for drinking purposes especially with the meals. Products like tobacco, bidi, cigarette, pan masala and zarda should be avoided. With water treatments, like hipbath, hot footbath and chest pack give considerable relief to the Asthma patients. In the state of attack hot footbath gives immediate relief.

Treatment of Asthma by Yogic Asanas is also immensely effective. Kunjala, Jala Neti, Sutra Neti and Vastra Dhauti may be practised everyday. After those first five exercises of Surya Namaskara, all exercises of Udara Shakti Vikasaka (Excepting Kunjala) may be followed. Urdhvagati and Engine Race are also beneficial in Asthma. Tadasana, Katichakrasana, Ashwathasana, Tanasana, Sarvangasana, Chakrasana, Bhujangasana, Dhanurasana, Vajrasana, Ushtrasana, Gornukhasana, Ardha Matsyendrasana. Malsyasana and Shavasana are useful in this disease. Kapalabhati, Bhastrika, Suryabhedi Pranayama, Uddiyana Bandha and Agnisara are also beneficial in this disease. Aromatherapy is another method that is specifically for small children. Four drops of benzoin and four drops of rosemary oil should be added to the child's bath daily. The massage oil should be made using three drops of benzoin and three drops of lavender oil and rubbed on the chest at regular intervals daily. Also, one can try using a vaporizer in the child's bedroom at night, with benzoin, pine and rosemary oils.

In the emergency department of asthma, doctors may use a capnography which measures the amount of exhaled carbon dioxide along with pulse oximetry which shows the percentage of hemoglobin that is carrying oxygen, to determine the severity of an asthma attack as well as the response to treatment. More recently, exhaled nitric oxide has been studied as a breath test that indicates the airway inflammation in asthma.

Current treatment protocols recommend prevention medications such as an inhaled corticosteroid, which helps to suppress inflammation and reduces the swelling of the coating of the airways, in case of anyone who has frequent need of relievers or who has severe symptoms. If symptoms persist, additional preventive drugs are also added until the asthma is controlled. With the proper use of preventive drugs, asthmatics can avoid the complications that often result from overuse of relief medications in asthma.

Beneficial Juices in Asthma: Apricot, lemon, pineapple, peach, carrot, radish and celery.

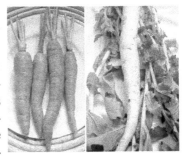

Horseradish and lemon juice: the potent ethers in fresh grated horseradish dissolve mucus in the sinuses and bronchial tubes quickly and effectively; mixing it with fresh lemon juice doubles its efficacy; grate fresh horseradish into a bowel, add enough fresh lemon juice to make a paste, take 1/2 tsp 2-3 times a day, as needed.

Carrot and radish juice: fresh raw radish juice is similar in effect to horseradish, but milder; it is too strong to take straight, however, and should be blended 5 oz with 11 oz carrot juice, 1 pint daily.

Cranberries: cranberries contain one of nature's most potent vasodilators, which open up congested bronchial tubes so that normal breathing is restored; cranberries are excellent curative and preventive therapy for the entire breathing apparatus; bring fresh cranberries to boil with just enough water to cover them, simmer 2-3 minutes, pour off excess water, puree cranberries in blender, strain off skins, and keep pulp in refrigerator; when asthma or other respiratory difficulty occurs, mix 2 tbsp in a cup of warm distilled water and sip slowly.

Chapter 8

Bronchitis

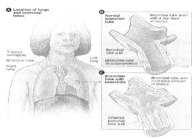

Bronchitis is inflammation of the mucous membranes of the bronchi, the airways that carry airflow from the trachea into the lungs. Bronchitis can be divided into two categories, acute and chronic, each of which has distinct etiologies, pathologies, and therapies.

Acute bronchitis is characterized by the development of a cough, with or without the production of sputum, mucus that is expectorated (coughed up) from the respiratory tract. Acute bronchitis often occurs during the course of an acute viral illness such as the common cold or influenza. Viruses cause about 90% of cases of acute bronchitis, whereas bacteria account for fewer than 10%.

Chronic bronchitis, a type of chronic obstructive pulmonary disease, is characterized by the presence of a productive cough that lasts for three months or more per year for at least two years. Chronic bronchitis most often develops due to recurrent injury to the airways caused by inhaled irritants. Cigarette smoking is the most common cause, followed by air pollution and occupational exposure to irritants.

Acute Bronchitis

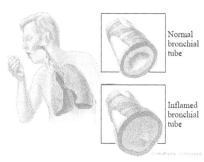

Normal bronchial tube

Inflamed bronchial tube

Acute bronchitis is most often caused by viruses that infect the epithelium of the bronchi, resulting in inflammation and increased secretion of mucus. Cough, a common symptom of acute bronchitis, develops in an attempt to expel the excess mucus from the lungs. Other common symptoms include sore throat, runny nose, nasal congestion (coryza), low-grade fever, pleurisy, malaise, and the production of sputum.

Acute bronchitis often develops during the course of an upper respiratory infection (URI) such as the common cold or influenza. About 90% of cases of acute bronchitis are caused by viruses, including rhinoviruses, adenoviruses, and influenza. Bacteria, including Mycoplasma pneumoniae, Chlamydophila pneumoniae, Bordetella pertussis, streptococcus pneumoniae, and haemophilus influenzae, account for about 10% of cases.

Treatment for acute bronchitis is primarily symptomatic. Non-steroidal anti-inflammatory drugs (NSAIDs) may be used to treat fever and sore throat. Decongestants can be useful in patients with nasal congestion, and expectorants may be used to loosen mucus and increase expulsion of sputum. Cough suppressants may be used if the cough interferes with sleep or is bothersome, although coughing may be useful in expelling sputum from the airways. Even with no treatment, most cases of acute bronchitis resolve quickly.

Only about 5–10% of bronchitis cases are caused by a bacterial infection. Most cases of bronchitis are caused by a viral infection and are "self-limiting" and resolve themselves in a few weeks. As most cases of acute bronchitis are caused by viruses, antibiotics should not generally be used, since they are effective only against bacteria. Using antibiotics in patients without bacterial infections promotes the development of antibiotic-resistant bacteria, which may lead to greater morbidity and mortality. However, even in cases of viral bronchitis, antibiotics may be indicated in certain patients in order to prevent the occurrence of secondary bacterial infections.

Chronic Bronchitis

Chronic bronchitis, a type of chronic obstructive pulmonary disease, is defined by a productive cough that lasts for 3 months or more per year for at least 2 years. Other symptoms may include wheezing and shortness of breath, especially upon exertion. The cough is often worse soon after awakening, and the spu-

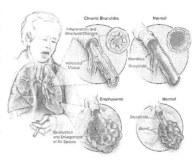

tum produced may have a yellow or green colour and may be streaked with blood.

Chronic bronchitis is caused by recurring injury or irritation to the respiratory epithelium of the bronchi, resulting in chronic inflammation, edema (swelling), and increased production of mucus by goblet cells. Airflow into and out of the lungs is partly blocked because of the swelling and extra mucus in the bronchi or due to reversible bronchospasm.

Most cases of chronic bronchitis are caused by smoking cigarettes or other forms of tobacco. Chronic inhalation of irritating fumes or dust from occupational exposure or air pollution may also be causative. About 5% of the population has chronic bronchitis, and it is two times more common in females than in males.

Chronic bronchitis is treated symptomatically. Inflammation and edema of the respiratory epithelium may be reduced with inhaled corticosteroids. Wheezing and shortness of breath can be treated by reducing bronchospasm (reversible narrowing of smaller bronchi due to constriction of the smooth muscle) with bronchodilators such as inhaled β-Adrenergic agonists (e.g., salbutamol) and inhaled anticholinergics (e.g., ipratropium bromide). Hypoxemia, too little oxygen in the blood, can be treated with supplemental oxygen. However, oxygen supplementation can result in decreased respiratory drive, leading to increased blood levels of carbon dioxide and subsequent respiratory acidosis.

The most effective method of preventing chronic bronchitis and other forms of COPD is to avoid smoking cigarettes and other forms of tobacco.

On pulmonary tests, a bronchitic (bronchitis) may present a decreased FEV1 and FEV1/FVC. However, unlike the other common obstructive disorders, asthma and emphysema, bronchitis rarely causes a high residual volume. This is because the air flow obstruction found in bronchitis is due to increased resistance, which, in general, does not cause the airways to collapse prematurely and trap air in the lungs.

Protracted Bacterial Bronchitis

Protracted bacterial bronchitis is defined as a chronic wet cough, with a positive bronchoalveolar lavage (BAL), that resolves with antibiotics. It is usually caused by streptococcus pneumoniae, haemophilus influenzae, or moraxella catarrhalis.

Treatment of Bronchitis by Nature Cure

Diet:

The patient should have one tablespoon of onion juice in the morning. He should also fast during the first two days by having orange juice mixed (with 50 percent water) every two hours for two days. This should also be followed by all fruit diet for another two days. He can also have water mixed with turmeric powder twice a day on empty stomach, also radish juice with water at least twice a day. Boiled concoction of ginger, black pepper and holy basil (Tulsi) should also be taken three times a day. The bronchitis patients should avoid soft drinks, refrigerated food, tea, and coffee, condiments, pickles and flesh foods.

Beneficial Juices in Bronchitis: Amla, Apricot, lemon, pineapple, peach, tomato, carrot, onion and spinach.

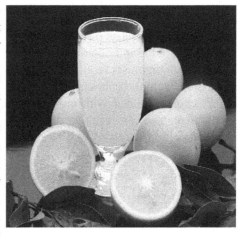

In acute cases of bronchitis, the patient should fast on orange juice and water till the symptoms subside. The procedure is to take the juice of an orange in a glass of warm water every two hours from 8 a.m. to 8 p.m. During this period, the bowels should be cleansed daily with a warm water enema. After the juice fast, the patient should adopt an all-fruit diet for two or three days.

In case of chronic bronchitis, the patient may adopt an all-fruit diet for five to seven days in the beginning of the treatment. In this regimen, he should have three meals a day of fresh juicy fruits such as apples, pears, grapes, grapefruits, oranges, pineapples, peaches and melons. Bananas, and dried or stewed or tined fruits should not be taken. For drinks, unsweetened lemon water or cold or hot plain water may be taken.

After the all-fruit diet, the patient should follow a well-balanced diet based on the three basic good groups, namely, seeds, nuts and grains, vegetables and fruits. The patient should avoid meats, sugar, tea, coffee, condiments, pickles, refined and processed foods, soft drinks, candies, ice cream and products made from sugar and white flour.

Certain vegetable juices have been found valuable in the treatment of bronchitis. The combined juice of carrot and spinach is especially beneficial. Formula proportions considered helpful in this combination are carrot 10 ounces and spinach 6 ounces to prepare 16 ounces or 1 pint of juice.

Chapter 9

Urinary Problems

The urinary tract is made up of the kidneys, ureters, bladder, and urethra. These organs work together to produce, transport, store, and excrete urine, the yellowish fluid that contains waste products removed from the blood. Urine contains the by-products of our body's metabolism, salts, toxins, and water. For instance, blood, protein, or white blood cells in the urine may indicate injury, infection, or inflammation of the kidneys. Glucose in the urine may be an indication of diabetes.

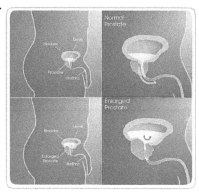

Problems in the urinary system can be caused by ageing, illness, or injury. As you get older, changes in the kidneys' structure cause them to lose some of their ability to remove wastes from the blood. Also, the muscles in your ureters, bladder, and urethra tend to lose some of their strength. You may have more urinary infections because the bladder muscles do not tighten enough to empty your bladder completely. A decrease in strength of muscles of the sphincters and the pelvis can also cause incontinence, the unwanted leakage of urine. Illness or injury can also prevent the kidneys from filtering the blood completely or block the passage of urine.

Some Diseases of the Urinary Symptoms:

Burning Urine

While passing urine some people feel burning sensation in the urinary passage. An infection in the urinary tract caused by diseases like gonorrhoea, enlargement of prostate, a stone in the urinary bladder or concentrated urine, as it happens in summer might be responsible for this type of complaint. Burning sensation may occur along with the passage of urine or may occur even after that. It may subside by taking some alkaline drinks or few glasses of water.

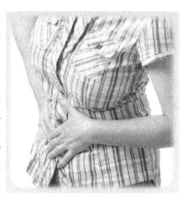

Hematuria
Presence of blood in the urine is called hematuria. According to Ayurveda it is a form of Adhoga Rakta Pitta. It is commonly caused by stones or infection in the genito-urinary tract and some other haemorrhagic conditions.

Nephritis
This refers to the inflammation of the kidney. It is of several types and in different stages of the disease it produces different types of symptoms. In Ayurveda it is called vrikka shotha.

Depending upon the variety of the nephritis, the signs and symptoms differ. Usually there is oedema in the face, which is more prominent in the morning and slowly subsides as the day passes on. The blood pressure may increase and the patient may suffer from biliousness, nausea, vomiting, abdominal pain, headache and diarrhoea.

Bed Wetting
It is the involuntary urination at night. Children after the age of 3 or 4 years normally possess sufficient control over their urinary sphincters in as much as they pass urine only when they want. Because of certain reasons, this control does not manifest because of which they continue to pass urine in bed at night. This continues in some cases, even up to the age of 15. Both boys and girls suffer from this ailment.

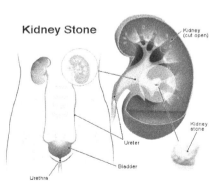

Kidney Stone

Kidney (cut open)

Kidney stone

Ureter

Bladder

Urethra

Kidney Stones
Urinary stones are generally formed by calcium, phosphates or oxalates. The main parts of the urinary tract are the kidney, ureter, bladder and urethra. The stones are formed primarily in the kidney and sometimes re-main there without being no-ticed for a long time. In certain circumstances they are slowly

dissolved or dislodged and come down, and during this process, they become lodged in a narrow part of the tract, giving rise to excruciating pain.

Stones are formed in the body because of vayu. It creates a type of dryness in the body because of which the chemicals start accumulating over the nucleus, that ultimately takes the shape of a stone. At times the entire kidney is filled with these stones and it becomes calcified and stops functioning. If urine is not excreted through the kidneys or excreted in small quantities, uremia sets in and causes many complications. The same phenomenon takes place if a piece of stone gets lodged in ureter or bladder.

The patient experiences pain in the lumber region of the kidneys at the back of the body.

Urinary Tract Infections

It is caused by bacteria in the urinary tract. Women get UTIs more often than men. Drinking lots of fluids also helps by flushing out the bacteria.

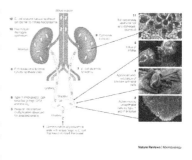

The name of the UTI depends on its location in the urinary tract. An infection in the bladder is called cystitis. If the infection is in one or both of the kidneys, the infection is called pyelonephritis.

Prostatitis

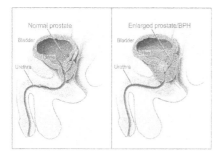

It is inflammation of the prostate gland that results in urinary frequency and urgency, burning or painful urination (dysuria), and pain in the lower back and genital area, among other symptoms. In some cases, prostatitis is caused by bacterial infection. But the more common forms of prostatitis are not associated with any known infecting organism.

Proteinuria

It is the presence of abnormal amounts of protein in the urine. Healthy kidneys take wastes out of the blood but leave in protein. Protein in the urine does not cause a problem by itself. But it may be a sign that your kidneys are not working properly.

Beneficial Juices in Urinary Problems/Bladder Ailments: Apple, apricot, lemon, cucumber, carrot, celery, parsley and watercress.

Fruit Juices that Affect the Urinary Tract

Fruit juices can be an important part of a healthy diet, but we may not always be thinking about the specific effects fruit juice can have on our bodies. Yet many fruit juices were once considered both a food source and a medicine. Fruit juices can affect the urinary tract in ways that are beneficial, but can also be less helpful in some situations.

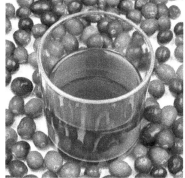

According to Medline Plus, urinary tract infection, also called UTI, is the generic term for an infection that may be in the bladder or kidneys. The terms cystitis, urethritis and pyelonephritis may also be used, depending on the actual location of the infection. Women are more likely to be infected than man, but diabetes, pregnancy or an enlarged prostate gland can also increase the chances of a UTI. Cranberry juice has been found to help prevent UTIs, although it will not cure an active UTI. According to naturopathic physicians Sally James and Nicholas Foley, members of the Australian Traditional Medicine Society, lemon juice will change the pH of the blood and urinary tract, which helps to prevent the bacteria that cause UTIs from growing.

Juice and Kidney Stones

Kidney stones are another urinary tract problem; the stones form from mineral crystals in the blood and can be very painful. Anahad O'Connor, a writer for the New York Times, noted in a March 2, 2010 article that fruit juices can be a two-edged sword when it comes to kidney stones. Cranberry juice, helpful in UTIs, also contains high quantities of oxalate, and can increase the chance of developing a kidney stone.

But citrus fruit juices, such as oranges, lemons and grapefruit, increase citrate levels and can help to prevent the formation of calcium oxalate stones --- the most common kind.

When to Use Fruit Juice

Your overall health history is important when considering the use of fruit juice for a particular kidney condition. If you have a history of both UTIs and calcium oxalate kidney stones, cranberry juice may not be a good choice for preventing UTIs. And diabetics should remember that fruit juices are high in natural sugars and can affect blood sugar levels. If you think fruit juice might be beneficial for you particular situation, it would be wise to discuss any questions or concerns with a health-care professional.

Hot spices are to be strictly avoided. The patient should be given as much water as possible to drink. Fresh lemon juice, fresh coconut water, orange juice, sugarcane juice and pineapple juice are extremely useful in this condition. The patient should be given fruits like apple, grapes, peaches and plums in good quantity.

The patient should not expose himself to sun or heat. Excessive perspiration takes away lot of water from the body and the urine thus becomes concentrated. Passage of this concentrated urine through the urinary tract causes irritation and gives rise to burning sensation.

Chapter 10
Common Cold

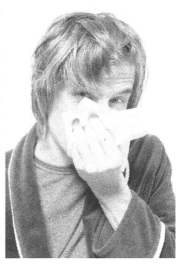

The common cold (also known as nasopharyngitis, rhinopharyngitis, acute coryza, or a cold) is a viral infectious disease of the upper respiratory system which affects primarily the nose. Symptoms include a cough, sore throat, runny nose, and fever which usually resolve in seven to ten days, with some symptoms lasting up to three weeks. Well over 200 viruses are implicated in the cause of the common cold; the rhinoviruses are the most common.

Upper respiratory tract infections are loosely divided by the areas they affect, with the common cold primarily affecting the nose, the throat (pharyngitis), and the sinuses (sinusitis). Symptoms are mostly due to the body's immune response to the infection rather than to tissue destruction by the viruses themselves. The primary method of prevention is by hand washing with some evidence to support the effectiveness of wearing face masks.

No cure for the common cold exists, but the symptoms can be treated. It is the most frequent infectious disease in humans with the average adult contracting two to three colds a year and the average child contracting between six and twelve. These infections have been with humanity since antiquity.

Signs and Symptoms

The typical symptoms of a cold include cough, runny nose, nasal congestion and a sore throat, sometimes accompanied by muscle ache, fatigue, headache, and loss of appetite. A sore throat is present in about 40% of the cases and a cough in about 50%, while muscle ache occurs in about half. In adults, a fever is generally not present but it is common in infants and young children. The cough is usually mild compared to that accompanying influenza. While a cough and a fever indicate a higher likelihood of influenza in adults, a great deal of similarity exists between these two conditions. A number of the viruses that cause the common cold may also result in asymptomatic infections. The colour of the sputum or nasal secretion may vary from clear to yellow to green and does not predict the class of agent causing the infection.

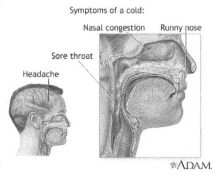

Symptoms of a cold:

Nasal congestion   Runny nose

Sore throat

Headache

✴ADAM.

Progression

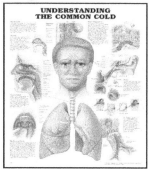

UNDERSTANDING
THE COMMON COLD

A cold usually begins with fatigue, a feeling of being chilled, sneezing and a headache, followed in a couple of days by a runny nose and cough. Symptoms typically peak two to three days after infection onset, and usually resolve in seven to ten days but some can last for up to three weeks. In children, the cough lasts for more than ten days in 35–40% of the cases and continues for more than 25 days in 10%.

Cause

Viruses

Coronaviruses are a group of viruses known for causing the common cold. They have a halo, or crown-like (corona) appearance when viewed under an electron microscope.

The common cold is a viral infection of the upper respiratory tract. The most commonly implicated virus is a rhinovirus (30–80%), a type of picornavirus with 99 known serotypes. Others include: coronavirus (10–15%), influenza (5–15%), human parainfluenza viruses, human respiratory syncytial virus, adenoviruses, enteroviruses, and metapneumovirus. Frequently more than one virus is present. In total over 200 different viral types are associated with colds.

Transmission

The common cold virus is typically transmitted via airborne droplets (aerosols), direct contact with infected nasal secretions, or fomites (contaminated objects). Which of these routes is of primary importance has not been determined. The viruses may survive for prolonged periods in the environment and can be picked up by people's hands and subsequently carried to their eyes or nose where infection occurs. Transmission is common in daycare and at school due to the close proximity of many children with little immunity and frequently poor hygiene. These infections are then brought home to other members of the family. There is no evidence that recirculated air during commercial flight is a method of transmission. However, people sitting in close proximity appear at greater risk. Rhinovirus-caused colds are most infectious during the first three days of symptoms; they are much less infectious afterwards.

Weather

The traditional folk theory is that a cold can be "caught" by prolonged exposure to cold weather such as rain or winter conditions, which is how the disease got its name. The role of body cooling as a risk factor for the common cold is controversial. Some of the viruses that cause the common colds are seasonal, occurring more frequently during cold or wet weather. Some believe this to be due primarily to increased time spent indoors in close proximity; specifically children returning to school. However, it may also be related to changes in the respiratory system that result in greater susceptibility. Low humidity increases viral transmission rates potentially due to dry air allowing small viral droplets to disperse farther and stay in the air longer.

Other

Herd immunity, generated from previous exposure to cold viruses, plays an important role in limiting viral spread, as seen with younger populations that have greater rates of respiratory infections. Poor immune function is also a risk factor for disease. Insufficient sleep and malnutrition have been associated with a greater risk of developing infection following rhinovirus exposure; this is believed to be due to their effects on immune function.

Pathophysiology

The symptoms of the common cold are believed to be primarily related to the immune response to the virus. The mechanism of this immune response is virus specific. For example, the rhinovirus is typically acquired by direct contact; it binds to human ICAM-1 receptors through unknown mechanisms to trigger the release of inflammatory mediators. These inflammatory mediators then produce the symptoms. It does not generally cause damage to the nasal epithelium. The respiratory syncytial virus (RSV) on the other hand is contacted by both direct contact and air born droplets. It then replicates in the nose and throat before frequently spreading to the lower respiratory tract. RSV does cause epithelium damage. Human parainfluenza virus typically results in inflammation of the nose, throat, and bronchi. In young children when it affects the trachea it may produce the symptoms of croup due to the small size of their airway.

Diagnosis

The distinction between different viral upper respiratory tract infections is loosely based on the location of symptoms with the common cold affecting primarily the nose, pharyngitis the throat, and bronchitis the lungs. There however can be significant overlap and multiple areas can be affected. The common cold is frequently defined as nasal inflammation with varying amount of throat inflammation. Self diagnosis is frequent. Isolation of the actual viral agent involved is rarely performed, and it is generally not possible to identify the virus type through symptoms.

Prevention

Physical measure to prevent the spread of cold viruses has been deemed the only potentially effective measure for prevention. These measures include primarily hand washing and face masks; in the health care environment, gowns and disposable gloves are also used. Efforts such as quarantine are not possible as the disease is so widespread and symptoms are non-specific. Vaccination has proved difficult as there are so many viruses involved and they change rapidly. Creation of a broadly effective vaccine is thus highly improbable.

Regular hand washing appears to be effective at reducing the transmission of cold viruses especially among children. Whether the addition of antivirals or antibacterials to normal hand washing provides greater benefit is unknown. Wearing face masks when around people who are infected may be beneficial; however, there is insufficient evidence for maintaining a greater social distance. Zinc supplementation may be effective at decreasing the rate of colds. Routine vitamin C supplementation does not reduce the risk or severity of the common cold, though it may reduce its duration.

Beneficial Juices in Common Colds: Lemon, orange, grapefruit, pineapple, carrot, onion, celery and spinach.

Juice Treatment

To treat a cold by means of customary suppressive drugs like aspirin and codeine only paves the way for future trouble of a more serious nature. For such a treatment puts a sudden stop to the eliminative process then taking place and forces the toxic matter back into the tissues again. Moreover, drugs have no effect on the duration of the cold. It has been aptly said that a cold can be cured in a week by taking medicines, otherwise it will subside in seven days.

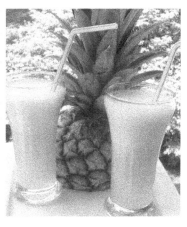

The only real treatment for colds is a proper diet. The best way to begin the treatment is to put the patient on a fast for two days. Nothing should be taken during this period except warm water mixed with lemon juice and honey or fruit juice and hot water. A liquid diet of fruit juice in large amounts is necessary to neutralizes the acid condition of the blood and hot drinks are needed to help clear the kidneys. Pineapple juice in particular is highly beneficial. A warm water enema should be used daily to cleanse the bowels during this period.

The short juice fast may be followed by an exclusive fresh fruit diet for three days. In this regimen, the patient should have three meals a day of fresh juicy fruits such as apples, pears, grapes, grapefruit, oranges, pineapple, peaches, melon or any other juicy fruit in season. Bananas, dried or stewed or tinned fruits, should not be taken. No other foodstuff should be added to the diet as otherwise the whole value of the treatment is lost.

After the exclusive fruit diet, the patient should gradually embark upon a well-balanced diet of three basic food groups, namely (i) seeds, nuts and grains (ii) vegetables and (iii) fruits. It is advisable to avoid meat, fish, eggs, cheese and starchy foods for a few days.

The patient should strengthen the system as a whole by taking a diet which supplies all the vitamins and minerals the body needs. Vitamin C, however, heads the list of these nutrients. It protects one against infection and acts as a harmless antibiotics. It is found in citrus fruits, green leafy vegetables, sprouted Bengal and green grams.

According to Dr. Linus Pauling, a noble prize-winning scientist, the regular use of this vitamin in the optimum daily amount will prevent the common cold and if a cold has already appeared, large doses of this vitamin will relieve the symptoms and shorten its duration. He estimates that one to two grams or 100 mg. to 200 mg. per day is approximately the optimum amount of this vitamin. His advice is to swallow one or two 500 mg. tablets of vitamin C at the appearance of first sign of the cold and continue the treatment by taking an additional tablet every hour.

Lime is the most important among the many home remedies for common cold. It is highly beneficial in all types of cold and fevers. It should be taken well diluted. Vitamin C-rich lime juice increases resistance, decreases toxicity and reduces the duration of the illness. Lime juice should be diluted in a glass of warm water, and a teaspoonful of honey should be added to it. It forms an ideal remedy for a cold and dry cough.

Chapter 11
Constipation

Constipation, difficulty in eliminating bowel movements from the body. Constipation is usually accompanied by the passage of hard, dry stools that may result in a tear in the lining of the lower rectum or anus or, more often, in painfully swollen and itchy veins in the lower rectum or anus, known as hemorrhoids. Tenseness and straining to achieve evacuation tend to worsen such conditions. Constipation is sometimes associated with feelings of sluggishness, headache, and distension of the abdomen.

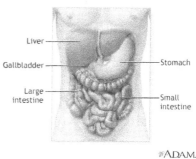

Chronic constipation may be caused by a diet insufficient in roughage or fibre, irregular eating hours, improper use of laxatives, or the voluntary avoidance of bowel movements. Many cases are believed to be caused by emotional disturbances. Constipation can usually be relieved by drinking adequate fluids; eating healthy foods such as fruits, vegetables, and cereals; and establishing routine evacuation habits. A high-fibre diet is particularly important for people who are taking medications that tend to harden stools and produce irregular bowel habits.

Some people become stressed or depressed when their bowel habits are irregular. Neglecting dietary measures, they may become addicted to the use of laxatives, suppositories, and enemas. These individuals may eventually lose muscle strength in the bowel wall, making it difficult for them to return to normal bowel habits. They also face the possibility that the digestive system will be unable to absorb all the nutrients in their food supply.

Constipation that develops suddenly in people who have previously had normal bowel function may be a symptom of a serious disorder, such as excessive production of thyroid hormones or kidney failure. Disturbing changes in bowel habits should be reported to a physician.

Treatment of Constipation by Nature Cure

Constipation is supposed to be the main cause of all diseases. Therefore it should be treated thoroughly. Several other disorders also crop up if the bowel is constipated like food digestion is delayed due to constipation. Food putrefies in intestine and results in Indigestion, Gas, Colitis, Pain in Abdomen, Backache, Appendicitis, Piles and Loss of appetite etc.

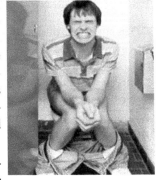

The first step in the treatment of constipation is to keep on fast for two to three days. During fasting lemon juice mixed with, honey in a glass of lukewarm water and lemon water enema should be taken daily morning.

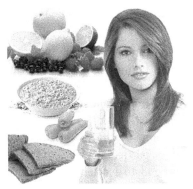

- ♦ If worms are present in the intestine then Neem water enema should be taken.
- ♦ The use of Castor oil is also advisable in the cases of chonic constipation.
- ♦ After completing the fast, fresh juice of juicy fruits should be taken and then shifted to fruit diet. Papaya, Pear, Guava and Figs are excessively helpful in removing constipation.
- ♦ After fruit diet Dalia and boiled vegetables and then gradually whole wheat bread and leafy vegetables should be started.

Food substances having more vitamin B are specially useful in removing Constipation.

♦ The patient must follow enema once or twice in a week according to the need even after the fast too.

♦ Light Sattvic Aahar should be taken after giving up the fried and heavy food substances.

♦ Before having a meal sufficient quantity of salad must be taken.

♦ Mudpack over abdomen and Hipbath of cold water is the excellent treatment of constipation.

♦ In the morning before going to the toilet a glass of cold water in summer and a glass of fresh water in winter may be taken. One should avoid purgatives because they are habit forming and the Natural mechanism of intestines become adversely affected due to it causing the chances of diseases like Piles, Prameha and Premature ejaculation.

♦ Morning walk is considered as a panacea for the patients of constipation if they improve their diet as prescribed above along with the walk.

Beneficial Juices in Constipation: Apple, pear, grapes, lemon, carrot, beet, spinach and watercress.

Prune Juice for Constipation in Infants

Most parents, especially the new ones, are worried about constipation in babies. Read on for more information about the use of prune juice for infant constipation

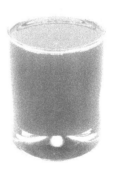

The bowel movements of a baby start with dark and sticky tar-like stools, which is called meconium. After a few days, the stools become mustard-coloured in case of breast-fed babies and tan-coloured in formula-fed babies. This is usually soft, seedy and runny. In general, the frequency of bowel movements in newborns is high, as they pass stools after every feeding. This frequency lessens as the baby reaches one month of age. As compared to formula-fed babies, breast-fed babies pass more stools per day. But some babies may not pass stools for several days and this condition is rare in exclusively breast-fed babies, as compared to formula-fed babies. A few days without any bowel movements is not a cause of worry, in case of infants. But if there is any other symptom, like irritability, vomiting or constant crying, you have to take your baby to a pediatrician immediately. For others, a few days without bowel movements is considered to be a normal condition, which may or may not amount to constipation in babies.

Infant Constipation

It is a misconception, that a baby who does not pass stools for more than two to three days, is suffering from constipation. As long as the stools are soft and watery, even if it happens at an interval or three or more days, it is not constipation. If the stools are very hard, dry and pellet-like and the baby is straining a lot to pass it, then the condition is called infant constipation which has to be identified by the parents. It is normal for an infant to grunt and strain while passing stools, but if he is experiencing constipation, he/she will strain more to pass the dry and hard stools. There can be bloating and loss of appetite too. Your baby may become irritable and may also have a tight abdomen. In some cases, there will be blood streaks in the hard stools, which causes anal fissures. This is a condition, which can be addressed with some exercises, massage, dietary changes and some home remedies. If you are looking for a home remedy for infant constipation, prune juice can be a good option.

Prune Juice for Constipation in Infants

This juice is manufactured by steaming prunes (dried plums) and then extracting the puree by putting them through a pulper. This extract is very high in fibre content and is popular for its laxative effect. It is one of the widely accepted home remedies for constipation. In case of infant constipation, prune juice is found to be very beneficial. It can be fed to babies, who are above the age of six months. Mix one ounce of this juice with one ounce of water and feed the baby, twice a day. This solution should be given to the infant, in addition to the daily food or breast milk. If you can make natural diluted juice, it will be much better. Otherwise, any regular bottled juice can be used, but make sure that the product is fresh, by checking the date of manufacture and expiry. Avoid adding sugar to the solution, which is made for the baby. This solution will loosen up the bowel and triggers bowel movement. In case of newborns and babies below the age of six months, consult your pediatrician regarding constipation remedies. It is always better to seek the opinion of your baby's doctor regarding the administering of prune juice for constipation in infants, even if your baby is above the age of six months.

Prune juice is an age-old home remedy for constipation in babies, but some babies may refuse to ingest it. In such cases, you may resort to other remedies, like baby massaging, warm baths and exercises like leg bicycling. Now that you know the benefits of prune juice for babies, you can try this remedy the next time your baby gets constipated.

Aloe Vera Juice for Constipation

Aloe Vera is a truly known medicinal plant which has been in continuous use for a period of about 1000 years for curing various type of diseases related to skin, herpes, burns, digestive system and many more. Aloe Vera juice is specially known to be used in curing several types of digestive and constipation ailments. Aloe Vera juice for

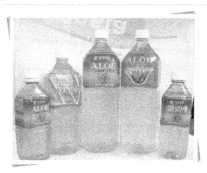

constipation is highly recommended for patients having stomach ailments and chronic gastro intestinal problems.

Aloe Vera Plants

There are several medicines to cure constipation but Aloe Vera juice for constipation is a natural remedy and is believed to be extremely beneficial. Aloe Vera acts as a stimulant laxative which when enters stomach helps in softening stools and makes the bowel functions normal.

Let us know how to use Aloe Vera juice for constipation and how it is beneficial for any type of stomach ailments. Firstly pure Aloe Vera gel is extracted from the plant and it is mixed with fruit juice. One should notice that the raw gel extracted directly from plant is more concentrated then that readily available in the market. So if you are using raw Aloe Vera juice for constipation then a quantity of about 5 ml is enough to be mixed with any fruit juice. Another option is to use Aloe Vera juice in the dry latex capsules which are readily available in any of the health shops. The most important thing is to follow the instructions about the manufacturer's dosage.

Aloe Vera juice for constipation can be used regularly if a person is suffering from chronic constipation ailment.

Also Aloe Vera juice which is used for helping constipation can be taken by gastro intestinal patients. Aloe Vera juice for constipation contains anti fungal properties that work to stimulate Candida and keeps the digestive track in tact. Aloe Vera juice for constipation can be taken with aloe Vera capsules along with turmeric or herbal tea so as to get better results and counteract the cramping which may accompany during passing stool.

Aloe Vera juice derived from the skin of Aloe leaf is a powerful laxative and contains almost 99 percent water, along with other substances known as glycol proteins and poly saccharine.

In some cases Aloe Vera juice for constipation is generally not recommended due to the fact of being laxative which in turn causes painful cramping. So it is not recommended to children below the age of 10 to take Aloe Vera juice for constipation. Else Aloe Vera is a very good medicine for curing almost all the stomach ailments.

Chapter 12

Colitis

Colitis, a chronic digestive disease and is characterised by inflammation of the colon. Colitis is one of a group of conditions, which are inflammatory and autoimmune that affects the tissue that lines the gastrointestinal system (the large and small intestine). Colitis is said to be an inflammatory bowel disease (IBD) and quite different from the irritable bowel syndrome (IBS).

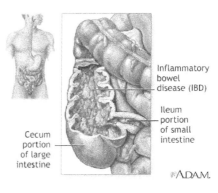

Inflammatory bowel disease (IBD)

Ileum portion of small intestine

Cecum portion of large intestine

＊ADAM.

The causes of colitis are also similar to that of Diarrhoea. The continuous intake of heavy, spicy food and the use of stale, polluted and adulterated substances, causes problems in the digestive system and it decomposes after reaching the intestines. Thus, the intestine fills up with stool due to non-cleansing of bowels causing the contamination of the Dhatus as well. However, natural efforts are made for this polluted matter to come out of the body. Sometimes, the urge of consumption of alcohol, change of atmosphere, consumption of cold food substances just after walking in sunshine and too much consumption of oily foods also causes Colitis.

Usually the signs and symptoms of colitis include pain, tenderness in the abdomen, depression, rapid weight loss, aches and pains within the joints, fatigue, changes in bowel habits in increased frequency, fever; swelling of the colon tissue, erythema or redness of the surface of the colon, ulcers on the colon in ulcerative colitis, which can bleed, mucus in the stool, blood in stool and rectal bleeding. Diarrhea can also occur, although some forms of colitis are constipation so the stool and bowel movements can appear normal.

Other symptoms of Colitis may include gas, bloating, indiges-

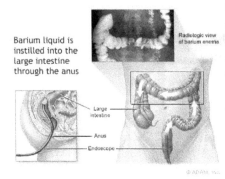

Barium liquid is instilled into the large intestine through the anus

Radiologic view of barium enema

Large intestine

Anus

Endoscope

tion, heartburn, reflux, Gastro oesophageal reflux disease, cramps, urgency and many other uncomfortable aches in the gastrointestinal system. Common tests, which reveal these signs of Colitis, include X-rays of the colon, testing the stool for blood and pus, sigmoidoscopy, and colonoscopy. Additional tests include stool cultures and blood tests, including blood chemistry tests. A high erythrocyte sedimentation rate (ESR) is one distinctive search in acute exacerbations of colitis. However, one or more types of foods can trigger the symptoms of Colitis.

The list of such triggers is as follows
- Caffeine
- Nuts, crunchy nut butters
- Alcohol
- Popcorn
- Carbonated beverages
- Seeds
- Dairy products, if lactose intolerant
- Spicy foods, sauces
- Dried fruits, berries, fruits with pulp or seeds
- Hot sauce, pepper
- Foods containing sulfur or sulphate
- Raw vegetables
- Dried beans, peas, and legumes
- Products containing sorbitol (sugar-free gum and candies)
- Foods high in fibre, including whole-grain products
- Refined sugar
- Spiders

Although there is little medical support for the idea, some people claim they have become completely symptom free by eliminating most foods; especially grains and other cooked foods, and are replaced by raw food diet based around fruits. Types of colitis include ulcerative colitis (UC), lymphocytic colitis, diversion colitis, Crohn`s colitis, chemical colitis, ischemic colitis, fulminant colitis, infectious colitis, collagenous colitis, microscopic colitis, and atypical colitis. A well-known subtype of infectious colitis is known as the pseudomembranous colitis, which results from infection by a toxigenic strain of Clostridium difficile, however parasitic infections can also cause colitis.

Any colitis with a speedy downhill clinical course is known as fulminant colitis. In addition to the diarrhea, fever, and anemia symptoms seen in colitis, the patient experiences severe abdominal pain and presents a clinical picture similar to that of septicemia, where shock is also present. Approximately half of these patients require surgery. Irritable bowel syndrome, a separate disease, has been called spastic colitis or spastic colon.

Treatment of colitis includes the administration of antibiotics and general non-steroidal anti-inflammatory (NSAIDS) medications such as Mesalamine (Asacol) or its derivatives; Azathioprine or similar immunosupressants; steroids such as prednisolone and prednisone; one or several of a number of other drugs that reduces inflammation and pain (buscopan). As it is a chronic condition the objective is "diminution" rather than cure. Surgery of Colitis is required only when the patient suffers from regular or permanent flare-ups, especially in cases of fulminant colitis. Surgery usually requires removing the colon and bowel and creating a "pouch" with a portion of the small intestine, which in time assumes the characteristics of the colon.

Medical opinion is classified on the basis of diet in colitis and IBD. Anecdotally, some sufferers find a change in diet and can be effective in treating the symptoms of colitis and easing the side effects. These include reducing the intake of complex carbohydrates, lactose products, refined sugar, soft drinks, caffeine, and spicy foods.

Treatment of Colitis through Nature Cure

Treatment of colitis through Nature Cure is said to be the best, buttermilk is very useful for colitis. Buttermilk may be prepared by mixing 4 times water in fresh curd and taken 3-4 times in a day, added with salt, jeera, heeng. But the curd should not be either too sweet or too sour. Hipbath is beneficial in this disease; however if not available, then even abdomen pack may be used for 30 minutes. Kati chakrasan is the apt Yogic Asana to treat colitis. The four naval correcting asanas may also be practised for the prevention of recurrent loose motions due to the displacement of naval towards lower side.

Beneficial Juices in Colitis: Apple, apricot, pear, peach, pineapple, papaya, carrot, beet, cucumber and spinach.

Papaya Juice

Naturopathy offers a natural cure for colitis. In the natural remedy, diet plays an important part in the treatment. At the initial stage, plain warm water with a little olive oil is consumed which is the only method of softening and removing the accumulations of hardened matter sticking to the walls of the colon. It is wise to observe a juice fast for five days or so in most cases of ulcerative colitis. The juices may be diluted with a little boiled water. Papaya juice, raw cabbage and carrot juices will be in particular beneficial. Citrus juices should be avoided. The bowel should be cleansed daily with a warm water enema.

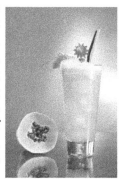

After the juice fast, the patient should gradually adopt a diet of small, regular meals of soft cooked or steamed vegetables, rice, dalia (coarsely broken wheat), well ripened fruits like banana and papaya, yogurt and home-made cottage cheese. Sprouted seeds and grains, whole meal bread and raw vegetables may be added gradually to this diet after about ten days. All food must be eaten slowly and chewed carefully. Foods which should be excluded from the diet are white sugar, white bread and white flour products, highly seasoned foods, highly salted foods, strong tea, coffee and alcoholic beverages and foods cooked in aluminium pans. Ripe bananas are highly advantageous in the treatment of ulcerative colitis, being bland, smooth, easily digested and slightly laxative.

Another valuable remedy for ulcerative colitis is the use of butter-milk. It is the residual milk left after the fat has been removed from yogurt by churning. Butter milk enema twice a week is also comforting and helps in re-installing a healthy flora in the colon. An effective cure for colitis is tender coconut water; it is soothing to the soft mucosa of the colon. Cooked apple also aids the healing of ulcerative conditions because of its sufficient concentration of iron and phosphorous. The patient should have a bowel movement at the same time each day and spend ten to fifteen minutes in the endeavour. Drinking two glasses of water the first thing in the morning will stimulate a normal bowel movement. An enema may be used if no bowel movement occurs. Complete bed rest and plenty of liquids are very essential. The patient should eliminate all causes of tension, adjust to his disability and face his anxiety with patience.

Banana Juice

Ripe bananas are a alkaline-forming food and one of the very few foods that contain all of the important vitamins.

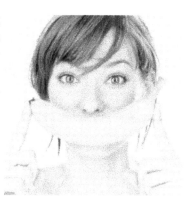

Banana is widely appreciated for its flavour and aroma (isoamyl lacetate) either as banana juice or a mixture with other juice.

To get the juice from bananas, cut them onto slices and soak them in water overnight. Then put them though the juice extractor with liquid, adding a teaspoon of lemon juice. Drink one pint daily.

Bananas have high sugar content and a recognizable, desirable flavour, high value clarified juices become a valuable product for drinking juice.

Normally, juice is consumed after dilution to acceptable sweetness. Acceptable sweetness has been established to coincide with a Brix of between 12% and 14%.

Banana juice has been known to ease the fissuring of people who have colitis and heartburn. It is an excellent source of potassium and vitamin A and a number of other beneficial elements.

Chapter 13

Diabetes

Diabetes Mellitus is a disease in which the pancreas produces insufficient amounts of insulin, or in which the body's cells fail to respond appropriately to insulin. Insulin is a hormone that helps the body's cells absorb glucose (sugar) so it can be used as a source of energy. In people with diabetes, glucose levels build up in the blood and urine, causing excessive urination, thirst, hunger, and problems with fat and protein metabolism.

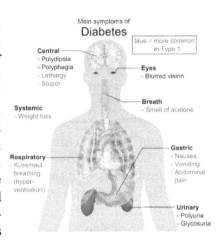

Main symptoms of
Diabetes

blue = more common in Type 1

Central
- Polydipsia
- Polyphagia
- Lethargy
- Stupor

Systemic
- Weight loss

Respiratory
- Kussmaul breathing (hyper-ventilation)

Eyes
- Blurred vision

Breath
- Smell of acetone

Gastric
- Nausea
- Vomiting
- Abdominal pain

Urinary
- Polyuria
- Glycosuria

Diabetes mellitus differs from the less common diabetes insipidus, which is caused by lack of the hormone vasopressin, which controls the amount of urine secreted.

In the United States, some 21 million people (7 percent of the population) suffer from diabetes mellitus. Every year, some 1.5 million people learn they have the disease. Diabetes mellitus kills more than 73,000 U.S. residents each year, making it the sixth leading cause of all deaths resulting from disease. In addition, diabetes is a contributing factor in many deaths from heart disease, kidney failure, and other conditions. Overall, experts estimate that diabetes contributes to about 225,000 deaths annually in the United States. In Canada, approximately 2.5 million residents (about 6 percent of the population) have diabetes mellitus. The disease ranks as the seventh leading cause of death in Canada, where it kills about 6,000 people a year. Diabetes and its complications contribute to about 25,000 deaths in Canada annually.

Diabetes is most common in adults over 45 years of age; in people who are overweight or physically inactive; in individuals who have an immediate family member with diabetes; and in people of African,

Hispanic, and Native American descent. The highest rate of diabetes in the world occurs in Native Americans. More women than men have been diagnosed with the disease.

In diabetes mellitus low insulin levels or poor response to insulin prevent cells from absorbing glucose. As a result, glucose builds up in the blood. When glucose-laden blood passes through the kidneys, the organs that remove blood impurities, the kidneys cannot absorb all of the excess glucose. This excess glucose spills into the urine, accompanied by water and electrolytes—ions required by cells to regulate the electric charge and flow of water molecules across the cell membrane. This causes frequent urination to get rid of the additional water drawn into the urine; excessive thirst to trigger replacement of lost water; and hunger to replace the glucose lost in urination. Additional symptoms may include blurred vision, dramatic weight loss, irritability, weakness and fatigue, and nausea and vomiting.

Type 1 Diabetes

Diabetes is classified into two types. In Type 1 diabetes, formerly called insulin-dependent diabetes mellitus (IDDM) and juvenile-onset diabetes, the body does not produce insulin or produces it only in very small quantities. Symptoms usually appear suddenly, typically in individuals under 20 years of age. Most cases occur around puberty—around age 10 to 12 in girls and age 12 to 14 in boys. In the 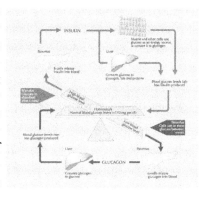 United States Type 1 diabetes accounts for 5 to 10 percent of all diabetes cases. In Canada, Type 1 diabetes accounts for about 10 percent of all diabetes cases.

Type 1 diabetes is an autoimmune disease, that is, a condition in which the body's disease-fighting immune system goes awry and attacks healthy tissues. In the case of Type 1 diabetes, the immune system mistakenly attacks and destroys insulin-producing cells, known as beta cells, in the pancreas. Scientists believe that a combination of genetic and environmental factors somehow triggers the immune system to destroy these cells. Scientists have so far identified 20 genes that play a role in Type 1 diabetes, although the exact function of these genes is still under investigation. Environmental factors, such as certain viruses, may also contribute to the development of the disease, particularly in people who already have a genetic predisposition for the disease.

In addition to causing a buildup of glucose in the blood, untreated Type 1 diabetes affects the metabolism of fat. Because the body cannot convert glucose into energy, it begins to break down stored fat for fuel. This produces increasing amounts of acidic compounds in the blood called ketone bodies, which interfere with cellular respiration, the energy-producing process in cells.

Type 2 Diabetes

In Type 2 diabetes, formerly known as non-insulin-dependent diabetes mellitus (NIDDM) and adult-onset diabetes, the body's delicate balance between insulin production and the ability of cells to use insulin goes awry. Symptoms characteristic of Type 2 diabetes include those found in Type 1 diabetes, as well as repeated infections or skin sores that heal slowly or not at all, generalized tiredness, and tingling or numbness in the hands or feet.

Of the nearly 21 million people in the United States with diabetes, 90 to 95 percent have Type 2 diabetes. About 90 percent of all diabetes cases in Canada are Type 2. The onset of Type 2 diabetes usually occurs after the age of 45, although the incidence of the disease in younger people is growing rapidly. Because symptoms develop slowly, individuals with the disease may not immediately recognize that they are sick. A number of genes are involved in Type 2 diabetes. In addition, there is a strong relationship between obesity and Type 2 diabetes. About 80 percent of diabetics with this form of the disease are significantly overweight.

Complications

If left untreated, diabetes mellitus may cause life-threatening complications. Type 1 diabetes can result in diabetic coma (a state of unconsciousness caused by extremely high levels of glucose in the blood) or death. In both Type 1 and Type 2 diabetes, complications may include blindness, kidney failure, and heart disease. Diabetes can cause tiny blood vessels to become blocked; when this occurs in blood vessels of the eye, it can result in *retinopathy* (the breakdown of the lining at the back of the eye), causing blindness. Diabetes mellitus is the leading cause of new cases of blindness in people aged 20 to 74. In the kidneys, diabetes can lead to *nephropathy* (the

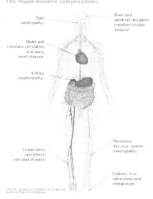

inability of the kidney to properly filter toxins from the blood). About 40 percent of new cases of end-stage *renal disease* (kidney failure) are caused by diabetes mellitus. Blockages of large blood vessels in diabetics can lead to many cardiovascular problems, including high blood pressure, heart attack, and stroke. Although these conditions also occur in nondiabetic individuals, people with diabetes are two to four times more likely to develop cardiovascular disorders.

Diabetes mellitus may also cause loss of feeling, particularly in the lower legs. This numbness may prevent a person from feeling the pain or irritation of a break in the skin or of foot infection until after complications have developed, possibly necessitating amputation of the foot or leg. Burning pain, sensitivity to touch, and coldness of the foot, conditions collectively known as neuropathy, can also occur. Other complications include higher-risk pregnancies in diabetic women and a greater occurrence of dental disease.

Diagnosis and Treatment

Diabetes is detected by measuring the amount of glucose in the blood after an individual has fasted (abstained from food) for about eight hours. In some cases, physicians diagnose diabetes by administering an oral glucose tolerance test, which

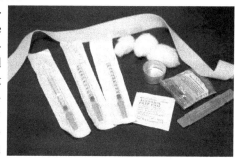

measures glucose levels before and after a specific amount of sugar has been ingested.

Once diabetes is diagnosed, treatment consists of controlling the amount of glucose in the blood and preventing complications. Depending on the type of diabetes, this can be accomplished through regular physical exercise, a carefully controlled diet, and medication.

Individuals with Type 1 diabetes must receive insulin, often two to four times a day, to provide the body with the hormone it does not produce. Insulin cannot be taken orally, because it is destroyed in the digestive system. Consequently, insulin-dependent diabetics have historically injected the drug using a hypodermic needle or a beeper-sized pump connected to a needle inserted under the skin. In 2006, the United States Food and Drug Administration approved a form of insulin that can be inhaled and then is absorbed by blood in the lungs.

The amount of insulin needed varies from person to person and may be influenced by factors such as a person's level of physical activity, diet, and the presence of other health disorders. Typically, individuals with Type 1 diabetes use a metre several times a day to measure the level of glucose in a drop of their blood obtained by pricking a fingertip. They can then adjust the dosage of insulin, physical exercise, or food intake to maintain the blood sugar at a normal level. People with Type 1 diabetes must carefully control their diets by distributing meals and snacks throughout the day so as not to overwhelm the ability of the insulin supply to help cells absorb glucose. They also need to eat foods that contain complex sugars, which break down slowly and cause a slower rise in blood sugar levels.

Although most persons with Type 1 diabetes strive to lower the amount of glucose in their blood, levels that are too low can also cause health problems. For example, if a person with Type 1 diabetes takes too much insulin, it can produce low blood sugar levels. This may result in hypoglycemia, a condition characterized by shakiness, confusion, and anxiety. A person who develops hypoglycemia can combat symptoms by ingesting glucose tablets or by consuming foods with high sugar content, such as fruit juices or hard candy.

In order to control insulin levels, people with Type 1 diabetes must monitor their glucose levels several times a day. In 1983 a group of 1,441 Type 1 diabetics aged 13 to 39 began participating in the Diabetes Control and Complications Trial (DCCT), the largest scientific study of diabetes treatment ever undertaken. The DCCT studied the potential for reducing diabetes-related complications, such as nerve or kidney disease or eye disorders, by having patients closely monitor their blood sugar levels four to six times a day, maintaining the levels as close to normal as possible. The results of the study, reported in 1993, showed a 50 to 75 percent reduction of diabetic complications in people who aggressively monitored and controlled their glucose levels. Although the study was performed on people with Type 1 diabetes, researchers believe that close monitoring of blood sugar levels would also benefit people with Type 2 diabetes.

For persons with Type 2 diabetes, treatment begins with diet control, exercise, and weight reduction, although over time this treatment may not be adequate. People with Type 2 diabetes typically work with nutritionists to formulate a diet plan that regulates blood sugar levels so that they do not rise too swiftly after a meal. A recommended meal is usually low in fat (30 percent or less of total calories), provides moderate protein (10 to 20 percent of total calories), and contains a variety of carbohydrates, such as beans, vegetables, and grains. Regular exercise helps body cells absorb glucose—even ten minutes of exercise a day can be effective. Diet control and exercise may also play a role in weight reduction, which appears to partially reverse the body's inability to use insulin.

For some people with Type 2 diabetes, diet, exercise, and weight reduction alone may work initially, but eventually this regimen does not help control high blood sugar levels. In these cases, oral medication may be prescribed. If oral medications are ineffective, a person with Type 2 diabetes may need insulin doses or a combination of oral medication and insulin. About 50 percent of individuals with Type 2 diabetes require oral medications, 40 percent require insulin or a combination of insulin and oral medications, and 10 percent use diet and exercise alone.

Current Research

At present no cure exists for diabetes, and scientists are unsure of the exact cause, although researchers are investigating a combination of genetic and environmental factors. So far researchers have identified 20 genes involved in Type 1 diabetes, and they are working to determine each gene's role in causing the disease. The inheritance patterns of Type 1 diabetes are complicated, with many different genes influencing a person's risk. For instance, a gene known as DR plays a role in Type 1 diabetes. Two forms of this gene, called DR3 and DR4, are present in 95 percent of people with Type 1 diabetes. People who inherit DR3 alone develop diabetes at an older age and have antibodies that destroy insulin-producing beta cells. Those who inherit DR4 tend to develop diabetes earlier in life and have antibodies that destroy insulin. A person with both DR3 and DR4 typically develops diabetes at a very young age and has the highest level of insulin-destroying antibodies.

In 2000 researchers were surprised to find that a variation of a gene called Caplain-10, which is not involved in glucose metabolism, is associated with the development of Type 2 diabetes. One form of this gene produces a small amount of protein, and researchers are studying how this decrease in protein increases a person's risk for diabetes. Other genetic studies indicate that certain genes cause a variation of Type 2 diabetes called maturity onset diabetes of the young (MODY), which develops in people under the age of 25. Although scientists do not yet understand how these genes cause MODY, the genes are known to be active in the liver, intestine, kidney, and pancreas.

Other scientists hope to identify the environmental factors that trigger Type 1 diabetes in people with a genetic predisposition for the disease. If they can determine what causes the immune system to attack the cells that produce insulin, they may discover how to prevent the condition from developing. For instance, studies suggest that certain viruses, such as coxsackie B, rubella, and mumps, may trigger an immune reaction against beta cells or in some cases directly infect and destroy these cells.

Researchers attribute most cases of Type 2 diabetes to obesity. Studies show that the risk for developing Type 2 diabetes increases by 4 percent for every pound of excess weight a person carries. Researchers are investigating the exact role that extra weight plays in preventing the proper utilization of insulin and why some overweight people develop the disease while others do not.

Research also focuses on transplanting a healthy pancreas or its insulin-producing beta cells into a person with Type 1 diabetes to provide a natural source of insulin. Some patients who have received pancreas transplants have experienced considerable improvements in their health, but positive, long-term results with beta-cell transplants have not yet occurred. In both types of transplants recipients must take drugs that suppress their immune systems so the body will not reject the new pancreas or cells. These drugs can cause life-threatening side effects because the patient's body can no longer protect itself from other harmful substances. In most people with diabetes, these drugs pose a greater risk to health than living with diabetes. Scientists are also studying the development of an artificial pancreas and ways to genetically manipulate non-insulin-producing cells into making insulin.

New methods for accurately measuring blood glucose levels may improve the quality of life for many individuals with diabetes. New techniques include the use of laser beams and infrared technology. For example, a tiny computer using infrared light can be used to measure a person's blood sugar level. The computer automatically delivers the reading to an insulin pump carried on the diabetic's body that injects the appropriate amount of insulin.

Other advances include new drugs that control blood sugar. In April 2000 the United States Food and Drug Administration (FDA) approved glargine, an insulin drug that needs to be injected only once a day. Sold under the brand name Lantus, this drug can be used by people with Type 1 diabetes, as well as by those with Type 2 diabetes who require insulin injections. And, as mentioned earlier, in 2006 the FDA approved a form of insulin that can be inhaled. Physicians have long known that some insulin-dependent diabetics fail to take the drug as often as needed because of the discomfort of injections. Doctors hoped the inhalant form of insulin would lead to better patient compliance.

A number of drugs have been developed to help people with Type 2 diabetes. Examples include acarbose, (sold under the brand name Precose), which controls blood sugar by slowing the digestion of carbohydrates; and metformin (sold under the brand name Glucophage), which controls liver production of sugar, causes weight loss, and reduces total cholesterol. Pioglitazone (brand name, Actos) and rosiglitazone (brand name, Avandia) are drugs that make the cells more sensitive to insulin.

Beneficial Juices in Diabetes: Citrus fruits, carrot, celery, lettuce and spinach.

How to Juice with Diabetes

If you are diabetic, be aware of how many carbohydrates you drink anytime you have juice, and adjust your medication or exercise accordingly to avoid spikes in blood glucose levels (BGL). The best kind of juice is the one you make yourself. Fruit juices are higher in carbs and thus spike BGL more than most vegetable juices, although there are exceptions, like carrots and beets.

Instructions

Check your blood sugar level before juicing. If it is high, fruit juice is not the best choice. A vegetable juice might work better. Consider that a 4 ounce orange juice, typically four oranges, contains 15 carbohydrates. Four ounces is a gulp. Usually we drink 8 or 12 ounces at a time. Adjust your medication and exercise accordingly to compensate.

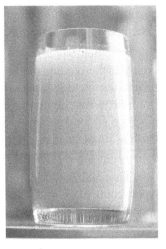

Chose the fruit you like and find out how many carbs you'll be taking in. Whenever possible use organic, clean fruits and use the peel, which adds fibre. The more fibre, the more balanced the impact on your BGL. Adding a tablespoon of flax seed meal increases the juice's fibre content. To minimize the impact on your BGL, add filtered water to the juice in your blender. Whole ginger adds spice and fibre, and it benefits your immune system.

If your BGL is low, drinking fruit juice is a good way to correct it.

Juice vegetables to make the most beneficial juice for diabetes. Leafy greens like kale, collard and mustard greens are high in fibre and very low in carbohydrates. Ginger adds spice and cleansing power to your juice. If you don't like to eat vegetables and salads, this kind of juice is perfect to add the nutritional value of vegetables to your diet.

Cucumbers are a good source of juice and low in carbs. Keep the peel to increase the fibre content.

Add garlic and/or onion if you like them. Onion helps lowering BGL, and garlic strengthens your immune system.

Combine vegetables and fruits. Vegetables are a good source of fibre; fruits taste good. Combine the two and you have a healthy juice beneficial for diabetes.

For example, juice together 1 cup of chopped kale (7 carbs), one whole cucumber (11 carbs), one medium size whole apple (17 carbs),

1/8 cup sliced ginger (2 carbs) and 1 tbsp. of flaxseed meal (2 carbs) for a total of 39 carbs. Add almonds or other nuts to make the juice more of a meal, with protein and fibre content.

Tips and Warnings
You can add flaxseed meal, oat bran, seeds and nuts to add taste, fibre and protein and reduce the impact on your BGL. Get creative.

Be aware of the impact that drinking juice has on your BGL and adjust your exercise and medication accordingly.

Juices That are Good for Type 2 Diabetics
Doctors will often advise their diabetic patients to avoid drinking sugary drinks, including fruit juice. In recent years, fruit juice manufacturers have responded to that admonition by producing lines of reduced-sugar juices that are more appropriate for type 2 diabetics. Certain vegetable juices and pomegranate juice may actually be beneficial for people with type 2 diabetes. If you have diabetes, check with your doctor prior to adding juice to your diet.

Pomegranate Juice
Pomegranate juice is filled with antioxidants, substances that help protect your cells from environmental damage and reduce your likelihood of developing heart disease, cancer and other chronic diseases. In the August 2006 issue of 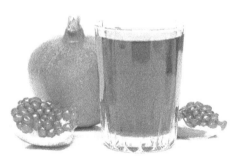 "Atherosclerosis," an article detailed the results of a study in which non-insulin-dependent diabetics drank 1.7 oz. of pomegranate juice daily for three months. Although pomegranate juice contains sugar, the participants in the study did not experience increases in their glucose, or blood sugar levels. The study included only 10 patients, however, so further research is needed.

Tomato Juice
Drinking tomato juice may improve the cardiovascular health of patients with type 2 diabetes. In a research letter published in the August 2004 issue of the "Journal of the American Medical Association," researchers

described a study that took place at the University of Newcastle in Australia. Participants with type 2 diabetes who supplemented with tomato juice over a three-week period experienced improvement in their blood platelet activity, reducing their risk of developing heart disease.

Fresh Juice

Purchasing a juicer allows you to have total control over the ingredients in your daily fruit or vegetable juice. In her book "Juicing Book: All You Need to Create Delicious Juices for Your Optimum Health," author Carole Jacobs, a former nutrition editor for "Shape" magazine, dedicates an entire chapter to diabetes and juices with a limited impact on blood glucose levels, including carrot, cauliflower-broccoli, cucumber and licorice root.

Chapter 14

Diarrhoea

Diarrhea, also spelled diar-rhoea, is the condition of having three or more loose or liquid bowel movements per day. It is a common cause of death in developing countries and the second most common cause of infant deaths worldwide.

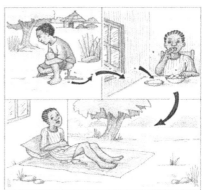

The loss of fluids through diarrhea can cause dehydration and electrolyte imbalances. In 2009 diarrhea was estimated to have caused 1.1 million deaths in people aged 5 and over and 1.5 million deaths in children under the age of 5. Oral rehydration salts and zinc tablets are the treatment of choice and have been estimated to have saved 50 million children in the past 25 years.

World wide in 2004 approximately 2.5 billion cases of diarrhea occurred which results in 1.5 million deaths among children under the age of five. Greater than half of these were in Africa and South Asia. This is down from a death rate of 5 million per year two decades ago. Diarrhea remains the second leading cause of death (16%) after pneumonia (17%) in this age group.

The following types of diarrhea may indicate further investigation is needed:

♦ In infants
♦ Moderate or severe diarrhea in young children
♦ Associated with blood
♦ Continues for more than two days
♦ Associated non-cramping abdominal pain, fever, weight loss, etc
♦ In travelers
♦ In food handlers, because of the potential to infect others;

♦ In institutions such as hospitals, child care centres, or geriatric and convalescent homes.

A severity score is used to aid diagnosis in children.

Diarrhea may be caused by bacteria
or parasites found in food and water

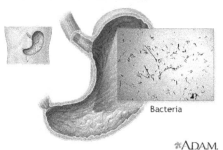

Bacteria

✵ADAM.

Osmotic

Osmotic diarrhea occurs when too much water is drawn into the bowels. This can be the result of maldigestion (e.g., pancreatic disease or Coeliac disease), in which the nutrients are left in the lumen to pull in water. Osmotic diarrhea can also be caused by osmotic laxatives (which work to alleviate constipation

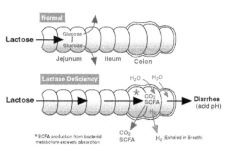

Fig. 2 Pathophysiology of Lactose Intolerance. SCFA = Short-Chain Fatty Acids.

by drawing water into the bowels). In healthy individuals, too much magnesium or vitamin C or undigested lactose can produce osmotic diarrhea and distention of the bowel. A person who has lactose intolerance can have difficulty absorbing lactose after an extraordinarily high intake of dairy products. In persons who have fructose malabsorption, excess fructose intake can also cause diarrhea. High-fructose foods that also have a high glucose content are more absorbable and less likely to cause diarrhea. Sugar alcohols such as sorbitol (often found in sugar-free foods) are difficult for the body to absorb and, in large amounts, may lead to osmotic diarrhea.

It can also be the part of the presentations of a number of medical conditions such as: Crohn's disease or mushroom poisoning.

Infections

There are many causes of infectious diarrhea, which include viruses, bacteria and parasites. Norovirus is the most common cause of viral diarrhea in adults, but rotavirus is the most common cause in children under five years old. Adenovirus types 40 and 41, and astroviruses cause a significant number of infections.

The bacterium campylobacter is a common cause of bacterial diarrhea, but infections by salmonellae, shigellae and some strains of "Escherichia coli" (E.coli) are frequent. In the elderly, particularly those who have been treated with antibiotics for unrelated infections, a toxin produced by "Clostridium difficile" often causes severe diarrhea.

Parasites do not often cause diarrhea except for the protozoan "Giardia", which can cause chronic infections if these are not diagnosed and treated with drugs such as metronidazole, and " Entamoeba histolytica".

Other infectious agents such as parasites and bacterial toxins also occur. In sanitary living conditions where there is ample food and a supply of clean water, an otherwise healthy person usually recovers from viral infections in a few days. However, for ill or malnourished individuals, diarrhea can lead to severe dehydration and can become life-threatening.

Malabsorption

Malabsorption is the inability to absorb food, mostly in the small bowel
but also due to the pancreas.

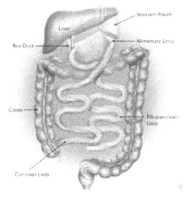

Causes include celiac disease (intolerance to wheat, rye, and barley
gluten, the protein of the grain), lactose intolerance (intolerance to milk
sugar, common in non-Europeans),
fructose malabsorption, pernicious
anemia (impaired bowel function
due to the inability to absorb vitamin
B12), loss of pancreatic secretions
(may be due to cystic fibrosis or pancreatitis), short bowel syndrome (surgically removed bowel), radiation fibrosis (usually following can-cer treatment), and other drugs, including agents used in chemotherapy.

Inflammatory Bowel Disease

The two overlapping types here are of unknown origin:

♦ Ulcerative colitis is marked by chronic bloody diarrhea and inflammation mostly affects the distal colon near the rectum.

♦ Crohn's disease typically affects fairly well demarcated segments of bowel in the colon and often affects the end of the small bowel.

Irritable Bowel Syndrome

Another possible cause of diarrhea is irritable bowel syndrome (IBS) which usually presents with abdominal discomfort relieved by defecation and unusual stool (diarrhea or constipation) for at least 3 days a week over the previous 3 months. There is no direct treatment for IBS, however symptoms can be managed through a combination of dietary changes, soluble fibre supplements, and/or medications.

Other Causes

♦ Diarrhea can be caused by chronic ethanol ingestion.

♦ Ischemic bowel disease. This usually affects older people and can be due to blocked arteries.

♦ Hormone-secreting tumors: some hormones (e.g., serotonin) can cause diarrhea if excreted in excess (usually from a tumor).

Diarrhea Treatment

A rotavirus vaccine has the potential to decrease rates of diarrhea. Research does not support the limiting of milk to children as doing so has no effect on duration of diarrhea.

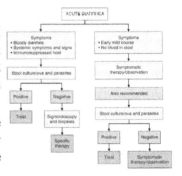

Medications such as loperamide (Imodium), bismuth subsalicylate may be beneficial, however they may be contraindicated in certain situations.

Medications

Antibiotics

While antibiotics are beneficial in certain type of acute diarrhea they are usually not used except in specific situations. In resource poor countries treatment with antibiotics may be beneficial.

Anti motility agents

Anti motility agents like loperamide are effective at reducing the duration of diarrhea. These agents should only be used if bloody diarrhea is not present.

Alternative therapies

Probiotics are bacterial supplements that can help prevent recurrence of diarrhea. The most widely used probiotics include lactobacillus and saccharomyces boulardii. For those who suffer from lactose intolerance, taking digestive enzymes containing lactase when consuming dairy products is recommended.

Beneficial Juices in Diarrhoea: Papaya, lemon, pineapple, carrot and celery.

Herbal Home Remedy for Diarrhoea using Mango : Mix ½ cup of sweet mango juice with 25 grams of curd and 1 tsp. of ginger juice. It cures chronic diarrhea, dyspeptic residue in diarrhea and piles.

Mosambi Juice

The acids present in the sweet lemon juice are great for doing away with toxins found in the bowel tracts. Mosambi juice is also beneficial for people with stomach upsets, dysentery, diarrhea and loose stools since it is rich in potassium. It helps avoid vomiting and nausea as a result of its tasty flavour.

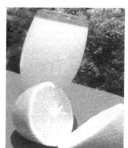

Chapter 15

Eczema

Eczema is a skin condition in which clusters of tiny elevated lesions are found that subsequently spread and coalesce into bigger patches. The disease affects persons of both sexes and at all stages of life. It is found to be hereditary in nature and has a preference for light-complexioned individuals and those 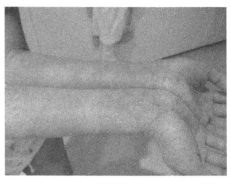 belonging to the economically backward class with poor nourishment. Proper hygiene, avoidance of allergens and exposure to the hot sun, intake of fruits and vegetables rich in vitamin C are necessary to prevent occurrence of the disease.

Symptoms of Eczema

Initially, eczema starts as localized reddening which later becomes edematous and scaly and subsequently oozes out serum. Thus, its symptoms can be listed down as follows:

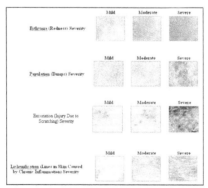

♦ Eruptions on skin

- Itching on the effected region
- Secretion of water or pus from the effected spot
- Red, rounded spots over skin
- Rough and thick skin surface

Causes of Eczema

The presence of any skin disease is like a warning to eliminate the morbid matter accumulated in the body by means of the skin. Usually such persons suffer from constipation and digestive disorders too. It is believed that eating abnormalities especially more consumption of sour, spicy, sweeter food items pollutes the blood by way of the Rasa produced from that food. This causes defilement of the entire blood stream. Pro-

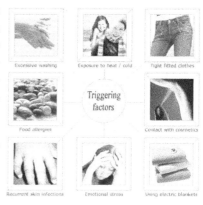

longed constipation is also one of the main causes of blood disorder. This contaminated and acidic state of blood is the cause of different types of skin disorders.

Treatment of Eczema by Nature Cure

Diet:

Skin diseases indicate that the internal system of the body is badly loaded with toxic substances and the body is being forced for eliminating the morbid matter through skin. Therefore, in its treatment, the internal cleansing method like fasting is an effective treatment. Short and long fasts are recommended according to the condition of disease and patient. Liquid diet for few days on juices rich in Vitamin C is also highly beneficial. Fruit and liquid diet may be taken instead of cereals while starting the treatment. During fast enema as well as bathing with Neem water (prepared after boiling Neem leaves) is highly beneficial.

Fruit and liquid diets gradually reduce the acidity, remedy the perverted stage of blood and help in restoring the normal healthy condition. In chronic skin diseases, fast should be done on water and after purification of body normal diet should be started, which includes whole wheat bread and green vegetables in sufficient quantity. Wheat Dalia and vegetables may also be taken. For getting rid of skin disorders however, sour, pungent, spicy and fried food substances should immediately be stopped.

Beneficial Juices in Eczema: Red grapes, carrot, spinach, cucumber and beet.

Epilepsy: Red grapes, figs, carrot, celery and spinach.

Spinach Juice

Raw vegetable juices, especially carrot juice in combination with spinach juice, have proved beneficial in the treatment of eczema. The formula proportions considered helpful in this combination are carrot 150 ml. and spinach 100 ml. to make 250 ml. of combined juice.

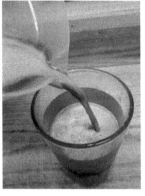

Vitamin-Rich Foods

According to Patrick Holford, author of "The New Optimum Nutrition Bible," the best diet for eczema is a vegan diet low in saturated fat and rich in essential fats. Holford recommends vitamins A and C to strengthen the skin, and vitamin E and zinc for wound healing. Eat foods rich in vitamins A and C, such as broccoli, tomatoes, watercress and melons. Obtain vitamin E and zinc from nuts, seeds and dark green leafy vegetables. According to "Alternative Medicine: The Definitive Guide," juice therapy may be beneficial for eczema. Cure this condition by using the combination of the following: black currants with red grapes; carrots, spinach, beets, cucumbers and parsley; wheat grass; and a variety of green juices.

Chapter 16

Gout

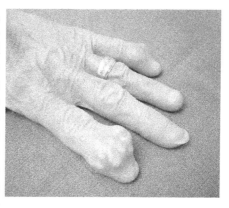

Gout, a metabolic arthritis, is a crystal deposition disease hallmarked by increased levels of uric acid (hyperuricemia) in the blood and causes inflammation. The condition holds that the crystals of monosodium urate (MSU) or uric acid are deposited on the articular cartilage of joints, tendons and surrounding tissues. It is marked by transient painful attacks of acute arthritis pioneered by crystallization of urates within and about the joints. It eventually leads to chronic gouty arthritis and the deposition of masses of urates in joints and other sites, which create tophi. Gout results from a combination of prolonged increase of uric acid and overall acidity in the bloodstream. In the ancient age, gout was called "the disease of kings" and "the king of diseases"; gout was recognised as one of the leading causes of painful, disabling, chronic arthritis.

There are some reasons that precede gout. The reasons include dietary imbalance, surgery and medicinal intake for some diseases. Among all these causes, fat is a common ingredient in the foods that cause gout. High intake of purine foods and dairy products can lead to gout. Even consumption of some vegetables like spinach, mushrooms, cauliflower, peas, asparagus, lentils and beans can accelerate gout. Earlier injury, surgery, high intake of alcohol, chemotherapy, even some diseases like Chronic kidney disease, High blood pressure, Hypothyroidism, Surgery and conditions that cause an abnormal rapid turnover of cells, such as psoriasis, multiple myeloma, hemolytic anemia, or tumors can direct to gout. The symptoms of gout are generally understood when one feels sudden onset of severe pain, tenderness, warmth, redness, and swelling from inflammation of the affected joint.

An attack of gout is usually accompanied by acute pain in the big toe, which becomes tender, hot and swollen in a few hours. The affected joints also become red, hot and painful. It may also similarly affect other joints such as the knees and the wrists, and sometimes more than one joint may be affected at a time. The attack usually occurs at midnight or in the early hours of the morning, when the patient is suddenly awakened. The acute attack generally lasts for a week or so. The disease may be accompanied by feverishness, vomiting and headache and also feel disinclined to eat. One's health, however, can also be aggravated by humid weather and errors in diet. If ignored, the disease can affect vital organs like the heart and the patient may suffer from palpitation and a sinking sensation.

The attacks are periodic and recur every few months and interval becomes shorter if the disease is not treated properly. The joint generally becomes damaged by arthritis. This is chronic gout, in which chalky lumps of uric acid crystals remain in the joint and also form under the skin. Another serious complication of gout is kidney stones containing uric acid, causing severe colic pains in the stomach in some cases the kidneys become damaged and do not function properly. This is a serious condition as the poisonous waste products, which are normally removed by the kidneys, accumulate in the blood.

In addition to that the increased level of uric acid in blood is also considered a symptom of gout. Gout usually affects a single joint and most often the big toe is affected. Gout is a disease resulting from the deposition of urate crystals caused by the overproduction or underexcretion of uric acid. Sometimes this disease is associated with elevated serum uric acid levels. Clinical manifestations include acute and chronic arthritis, tophi, interstitial renal disease and uric acid nephrolithiasis. The diagnosis is based on the identification of uric acid crystals in joints, tissues or body fluids. Detection of Hyperuricemia (high level of uric acid in the blood), Uric acid crystals in joint fluid are also taken as the symptoms of gout.

Heredity is another important factor in causing this disease and certain races are prone to gout. Other causes include regular eating of foods rich in protein and carbohydrate and lack of proper exercise. Stress is also regarded as an important cause of gout. During the alarm reaction, millions of body cells are destroyed and large quantities of uric acid freed from these cells enter the tissues after being neutralised by sodium.

There are different types of gout that include Asymptomatic hyperuricemia which is an early stage without any symptoms. Another type is Podagra which occurs in the big toe. About 75% of cases are found suffering from this type of gout. Acute gout is also named as acute gouty arthritis. Intercritical gout is another type of gout which is the symptom-free stage between attacks of acute gout. Chronic tophaceous gout is the most advanced stage of gout.

Treatment

Naturopathy prescribes proper intake of foods and balanced diet. The cure of gout needs to follow simple balanced food with minimum of proteins sub-stances and physical exercises. For an acute attack, the patient necessarily has to keep a fast for about five to seven days on orange juice and water. Sometimes the condition may worsen in the early stages of fasting when uric acid, dissolved by juices, is thrown into the bloodstream for elimination. This usually clears up if fasting is continued.

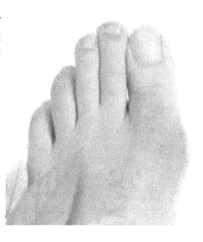

In severe cases, it is advisable to undertake a series of short fasts for three days or so rather than one long fast. A warm water enema should be used daily during the period of fasting to cleanse the bowels. After the acute symptoms of gout have subsided, the patient may adopt an all-fruit diet comprising three meals a day. The people who are suffering from acute gout or have diagnosed some symptoms of gout are advised to intake fruits such as oranges, apples, figs, apricot mangoes, whole wheat bread or `dalia` and milk or butter-milk. The patients are suggested to consume steamed vegetables such as lettuce, beets, celery water-cress, turnips, squash, carrots, tomatoes, cabbage and potatoes, `chappatis` of whole wheat flour, cottage cheese and butter-milk. Sprouts such as alfalfa and `mung` beans, a good-sized salad of raw vegetables such as carrots, cabbage, tomatoes, whole wheat bread and butter are good for the people suffering from gout.

The patient should avoid all purine and uric acid producing foods such as all meats, eggs, and fish. Glandular meats are especially harmful. Intoxicating liquors, tea, coffee, sugar, white flour and its products, and all canned and processed foods are harmful in such cases. Spices and salts should be used as little, as possible. Foods high in potassium such as potatoes, bananas, leafy green vegetables, beans and raw vegetable juices are protective against gout.

In alternative medicines, gout is treated by Water therapy. The treatment involves using some salts that should be used while bathing the affected areas. The feet should be bathed in Epsom salt foot baths twice daily. Half a pound to one pound of salt may be added to a foot bath of hot water. Full Epsom salt baths should also be taken three times a week. The baths may be reduced to two per week later. Cold packs at night, applied to the affected joints, will be beneficial. Fresh air and outdoor exercise are also essential. The patient should eliminate as much stress from his life as possible.

Beneficial Juices in Gout: Red sour cherries, pineapple, tomato, cucumber, beet, carrot, celery and spinach.

How to Treat Gout using Cherry Juice

Gout is a medical condition which attacks the feet and toes, making them swell and inflamed. It can start suddenly and it can be decapitating. According to research, the number of men who suffer from gout is higher than the number of women. There are different types of medical remedies including prescribed drugs and natural remedies as well which give the same benefits. The cherry juice is a common natural remedy for treating gout and it also helps in relieving pain and other symptoms.

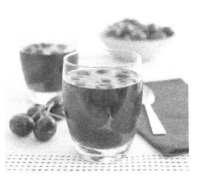

For those who are suffering from gout, drinking cherry juice is beneficial. The drink is made from dark red cherry and it contains a generous amount of vitamins and also minerals. It has been known to also contain anthocyanins, flavonoids and antioxidants. All these constituents make cherry juice a great cure for easing pain that is associated with gout. The anthocyanin pigment is what gives the berries the deep red colour which also contains anti- inflammatory elements. Cherry juice does help in the reduction of excessive uric acid that is in the blood stream which is the main cause of gout condition.

So as to gain the maximum benefits of drinking cherry juice, take two to three glasses of natural cherry juice each day. This is the same as consuming half pound of canned or fresh cherries and this will prevent any gout attacks. The cheery juice to be consumed is equal to 2 litres each day and it has to be pure for it to be effective. Drinking the cherry juice or even eating the cherries raw has the same beneficial effect on the body and in treating gout. They both have the same qualities although the juice may be easier to consume and is more affordable compared to the berries themselves.

Treating gout using cherries does not have any side effects unless if the patient is allergic to the black cherries. The body may need some time to get used to the idea of drinking this amount of juice but will soon get used to it. So a s to have a variety, mix the juice with any other dark berries like blackberries and raspberries which are said to contain similar beneficial properties in combating the pain and the symptoms that are associated with gout condition.

Chapter 17
High Blood Pressure

Hypertension or High Blood Pressure, medical condition in which constricted arterial blood vessels increase the resistance to blood flow, causing an increase in blood pressure against vessel walls. The heart must work harder to pump blood through the narrowed arteries. If the condition persists, damage to the heart and blood vessels is likely, increasing the risk for stroke, heart attack, and kidney or heart failure. Often called the "silent killer," hypertension usually causes no symptoms until it reaches a life-threatening stage.

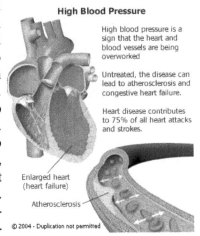

High Blood Pressure

High blood pressure is a sign that the heart and blood vessels are being overworked

Untreated, the disease can lead to atherosclerosis and congestive heart failure.

Heart disease contributes to 75% of all heart attacks and strokes.

Enlarged heart (heart failure)

Atherosclerosis

© 2004 - Duplication not permitted

Hypertension affects 20 percent of people living in the United States. Of these, almost a third are unaware of their condition. Until the age of 55, more men than women have hypertension. After that age, the condition becomes more prevalent in women. Hypertension is significantly more common in African Americans of both sexes than in other racial or ethnic groups.

Physicians use two measurements to describe blood pressure. Systolic pressure measures blood pressure as the heart contracts to pump out blood. Diastolic pressure measures blood pressure as the heart relaxes to allow blood to flow into the heart. An instrument called a sphygmomanometre measures systolic and diastolic pressure using units of millimetres of mercury (abbreviated mm Hg).

Blood pressure is classified in four categories: normal, prehypertension, stage 1 hypertension, and stage 2 hypertension. Normal blood pressure in an adult is less than 120/80 mm Hg, in which

120 describes systolic pressure and 80 describes diastolic pressure. Prehypertension is defined as a systolic pressure of 120 to 139 mm Hg or a diastolic pressure of 80 to 89 mm Hg. People with prehypertension are likely to develop hypertension at some point during their life. Stage 1 hypertension is defined as a systolic pressure of 140 to 159 mm Hg or a diastolic pressure of 90 to 99 mm Hg. Stage 2 hypertension is defined as 160/100 mm Hg or higher.

How Hypertension Develops

Two factors determine blood pressure: the amount of blood the heart pumps and the diametre of the arteries receiving blood from the heart. When the arteries narrow, they increase the resistance to blood flow. The heart works harder to pump more blood to make sure the same amount of blood circulates to all the body tissues. The more blood the heart pumps and the smaller the arteries, the higher the blood pressure.

The kidneys play a major role in the regulation of blood pressure. Kidneys secrete the hormone renin, which causes arteries to contract, thereby raising blood pressure. The kidneys also control the fluid volume of blood, either by retaining salt or excreting salt into urine. When kidneys retain salt in the bloodstream, the salt attracts water, increasing the fluid volume of blood. As a higher volume of blood passes through arteries, it increases blood pressure.

Scientists do not fully understand the causes of hypertension. In up to 95 percent of cases no clear cause can be identified. This type of high blood pressure is known as essential hypertension, and scientists suspect that genetic factors may play a role in its development. In about 5 percent of cases high blood pressure develops as a result of another medical disorder, such as kidney or liver disease, or as a side effect of certain medications. This type of high blood pressure is known as secondary hypertension. Other factors that may contribute to elevated blood pressure in some people include a diet high in salt, physical inactivity, obesity, and heavy alcohol consumption.

Complications

If hypertension is not detected and treated, life-threatening complications develop over a course of years. Increased pressure on the inner walls of blood vessels makes the vessels less flexible over time and more vulnerable to the buildup of fatty deposits in a process known as atherosclerosis. Weakened portions of the blood vessel wall may

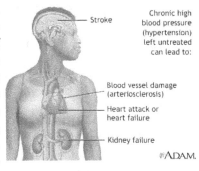

balloon, forming an aneurysm. If an aneurysm ruptures, internal hemorrhaging (bleeding) results. Both atherosclerosis and a ruptured aneurysm in the brain can lead to a stroke.

Hypertension forces the heart to work harder to pump adequate blood throughout the body. This extra work causes the muscles of the heart to enlarge, and eventually the enlarged heart becomes inefficient in pumping blood. An enlarged heart may lead to heart failure, in which the heart can not pump enough blood to meet the body's needs.

Increased blood pressure may damage the small blood vessels within the kidney. The kidney then becomes unable to filter blood efficiently, and waste products may build up in the blood in a condition known as uremia. Without medical treatment, kidney failure will result.

Treatment

Physicians recommend that people with prehypertension undergo diet and lifestyle changes, such as losing weight and quitting smoking, in order to prevent a rise in blood pressure. Some patients can lower their blood pressure by limiting salt in their diet. Increasing physical activity and reducing alcohol consumption to less than two drinks per day for men and one drink per day for women may also lower blood pressure.

For those with stage 1 and stage 2 hypertension, a physician may prescribe diet and lifestyle changes, as well as one or more drugs known as antihypertensives. Diuretics are antihypertensives that promote excess salt and water excretion, reducing the amount of fluid in the bloodstream and relieving pressure on blood vessel walls. Beta blockers reduce heart rate and the amount of blood the heart pumps. ACE inhibitors prevent the narrowing of blood vessel walls to control blood pressure. Calcium channel blockers slow heart rate and relax blood vessels. Studies show that two drugs are more effective than one drug at lowering blood pressure to less than 140/90 mm Hg.

Beneficial Juices in High Blood Pressure: Grapes, orange, cucumber, carrot and beet.

Celery Juice Every Day Keeps High Blood Pressure at Bay

Blood pressure is the force exerted by blood pushing against the walls of one's arteries. If the pressure rises significantly and remains there for an extended period of time, it can cause damage to the body. Lucky for us, one of the most common vegetables we use today - celery - with its stringy stems and crisp texture pro-

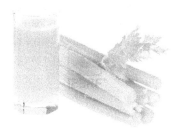

vides a natural way to lower blood pressure. It decreases a potentially dangerous situation without the risk of possible side effects that might accompany prescribed medication.

A blood pressure reading is measured by two numbers. The top number referred to as systolic is the measure of pressure the blood exerts while the heart is beating. The lower number, diastolic, is the measure of pressure the blood exerts while the heart is relaxed. The suggested optimal blood pressure is 120/80.

Just how could celery juice affect this measurement? This versatile veggie contains active compounds named phthalides. These compounds provide health benefits by naturally relaxing the muscles in and around the walls of the arteries which cause those vessels to dilate, creating more space inside the arteries that permits the blood to flow at a lower pressure. Phthalides also have been reported to lower blood pressure and promote a healthy circulatory system by reducing what are known as stress hormones. This biennial vegetable also contains high amounts of magnesium, potassium, and calcium. The beneficial effect of these minerals in celery serves to calm the nervous system, automatically counterbalancing stress levels.

Although Hippocrates (a Greek physician considered the Father of Medicine, c. 460 BC - c. 377 BC) prescribed the juice of this leafy-topped stalk to patients suffering from nervous tension and although Chinese medicine has long recognized celery juice to reduce high blood pressure, only recently has it been studied in the Western world.

The University of Chicago Medical Centre (UCMC) is credited with one of the first studies of celery's effects on blood pressure. In one instance, the father of a scientist at UCMC experienced a drop in his blood pressure from 158/96 to 118/82 after just one week of eating about four stalks a day.

To test this theory, a physician at the Whitaker Wellness Centre and her father both drank celery juice for thirty days, mixing it with a little orange juice to camouflage the slightly bitter taste of juiced celery. Their results? The father's systolic level dropped from 148 to 128, and the physician's went from 120 to 105.

Including this most nutritious juice as a part of a healthy diet and lifestyle just may help keep the risks of high blood pressure from ever becoming an issue.

Chapter 18

Halitosis

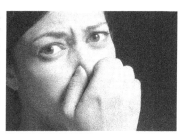

Halitosis refers to bad breath, which is a sign of ill health. It is very common disorder and is found in many people. Unfortunately, people who suffer from this disease are completely unaware of their problem and the discomfort they cause to others.

Causes of Halitosis

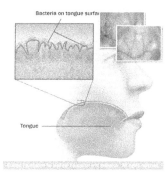

♦ The most common cause of halitosis is bad teeth and gum conditions. Dental decay at the roots of the teeth may result in abscesses in the gums with foul-smelling pus giving an objectionable odour to the breath. Even small holes in the teeth may provide a place where germs can multiply and release foul odour.

♦ Any conditions of the nose, throat, respiratory tract, or stomach which are associated with chronic infection or local upsets of one sort or another, such as chronic tonsillitis, lung diseases like chronic bronchitis and bronchiectasis, chronic gastritis and sinuses which cause a discharge at the back of the throat can be other causes of halitosis.

♦ Most cases of bad breath, however, are caused by gastro-intestinal disorders, intestinal sluggishness and particularly by chronic constipation. The unpleasant odour results from an exceptionally large amount of waste matter expelled through the lungs.

♦ Chewing pan, tobacco and smoking are also the other causes of bad breath. Diseases like anaemia may also lead to unpleasant breath.

Treatment of Halitosis by Nature Cure
Diet

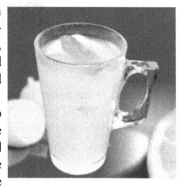

♦ The patients suffering from halitosis should take a well-balanced diet consisting of seeds, nuts, grains, vegetables and fruits, with emphasis on raw and cooked vegetables and fruits.

♦ All measures should be adopted to treat constipation if it is the cause for halitosis. The patient should avoid refined carbohydrate foods, such as white sugar, white bread and products made from them as well as flesh foods and egg. Even whole grain bread should be eaten sparingly.

♦ The patient should also avoid overeating. He should eat six to eight soaked prunes and a few dried and soaked figs with breakfast. He must also drink the water in which these fruits were soaked. He should also take plenty of liquids and drink six to eight glasses of water daily. This will help eliminate bad breath.

♦ All fruit and vegetable juices are beneficial in the treatment of halitosis and should be taken liberally by those suffering from this disorder. Juices from fruits like apple, grapefruit, lemon, pineapple and vegetables like tomato, carrot and celery are especially beneficial.

Home Remedies

Among the several home remedies for halitosis, the use of Fenugreek has proved most effective. A tea made from the seeds of the vegetable should be taken regularly for correcting the condition. This tea is prepared by putting a teaspoon of seeds in half a litre of cold water and allowing it to simmer for 15 minutes over a low flame. It should then be strained and used as tea.

The teeth should be cleaned regularly twice a day especially before going to bed at night. Meat particles should be removed carefully with toothpicks. In case of decaying teeth and swollen and bleeding gums, a dentist should be consulted. The use of twigs of the margosa tree as toothbrush is the best method of cleaning the teeth.

Another effective remedy for bad breath is the use of Avocado, which is far superior to any mouth lotion or remedies for this condition. It effectively removes intestinal putrefaction or decomposition, which is one of the most important causes of bad breath.

Munching a raw Apple or Guava after lunch removes most of the trapped particles in the mouth. The unripe guava hence, is useful in halitosis. It is rich in tannic, malic, oxalic and phosphoric acids as well as calcium, oxalate and manganese. Chewing it is an excellent tonic for the teeth and gums. It helps cure bleeding from gums due to styptic effect and stops bad breath. Chewing tender leaves of guava tree so stops bleeding from gums and bad breath.

Parsley is valuable in the treatment of bad breath. Two cups of water should be boiled and several sprigs of parsley coarsely chopped should be steeped in this water along with two or three whole cloves or a quarter spoon of ground cloves. This mixture should then be stirred occasionally while cooling. It should then be strained and used as mouths wash or gargle several times a day.

The person suffering from bad breath should take plenty of exercise, as lack of sufficient exercise is one of the main causes of constipation leading to halitosis.

Beneficial Juices in Halitosis: Apple, grapefruit, lemon, pineapple, tomato, carrot, celery and spinach.

Chapter 19

Headache

Headaches afflict almost everyone at some time or the other, since during most of the times, they are functional, caused by temporary upsets and are not related to any organic changes in the brain. A headache arises from irritation to nerve endings in the shoulder, neck and scalp muscles and also in the

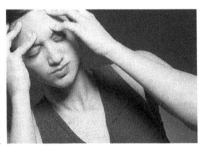

smooth muscles encircling the blood vessels, which serve these areas.

The Causes of Headaches

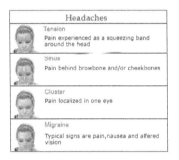

Poisons and toxins admitted into the body through food, beverages and water, as well as through breathing polluted air, can cause any number of disturbances. A headache may be the first warning that a poison has entered the body. Additives in foods and in many cases, cosmetics, skin and hair products are also serious offenders in bringing on headaches. In addition, there are many toxic air contaminants also that accumulate in the body, resulting in headaches.

The common causes of headaches are allergy, emotional reasons, eyestrain, high blood pressure, hangover, infection, low blood sugar, nutritional deficiency, tension, the presence of poisons and toxins in the body, and migraine. Intense emotion often causes headaches. This hidden hostility may manifest itself bottled as headache. It is important, therefore, that negative feelings should not be up, but should find some safe means of expression.

Eyestrain is a common cause of headache. In such cases, an eye specialist should be consulted and proper treatment taken thereon. High blood pressure can cause pounding headaches. The headache usually starts at the back of the head on getting up in the morning. Many people get a severe headache after consuming alcohol in excess. Alcohol causes the blood vessels to swell, resulting in a painful headache.

Headaches may occur if there is an infection, such as a cold, virus and fever also. Low blood sugar is one of the causes of irritability and headache. Low blood sugar is the result of an abused pancreas, which over stimulates the production of insulin in the body. Headache can also happen due to the deficiency of B vitamins, namely pantothenic acid, B-1 (thiamine), B-12 and B-6 (pyridoxine).

A lack of iron, resulting in anaemia, is a common cause of headache. The headache sometimes appears before the onset of anaemia, due to a chronic iron deficiency. Tension headaches are probably the most common of all, and are caused by emotional conflicts, which result in stress. Stress causes the muscles of the shoulder, neck and scalp to tense unconsciously. Persons who are irritable, tense and lose their temper quickly usually get this type of headache. It increases gradually and passes off with the release of tension.

Treatment for Headache by Nature Cure

Exercises

Since eyestrain always causes headaches, simple eye exercises should be practised to relieve eyestrain, such as moving the eyes up and down from side to side, palming, rotating the head with neck outstretched, forward and backward three times, then thrice clockwise and thrice anti-clockwise.

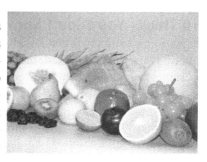

Water Treatment

A safe method of high blood pressure treatment for this is to immerse your legs to calf-level in a tub of hot water for 15 to 20 minutes. This draws the blood away from the head and down to the feet, giving relief from the headache.

Diet

The problem of headaches due to low blood pressure can be controlled by eating smaller meals at short intervals rather than the standard three large meals daily- The intake of carbohydrates should be cut down to the minimum and coffee should be eliminated as it over stimulates the pancreas.

Medicines

The best treatment for a headache after a lot of alcohol consumption is to avoid excessive consumption of alcohol. A hangover headache can be avoided by taking vitamin B-1 (thiamine) tablets with the drink.

If there is an infection, such as a cold, virus and fever then the headaches out of these disorders can be tackled. Vitamin C therapy is the best all-round method and for cold, since it's a natural antibiotic medicine. High doses should be taken at hourly intervals with the appearance of the first symptoms like a sore throat, runny nose, etc.

Brewer's yeast is an excellent source of iron and taking a few teaspoons daily can easily prevent anaemia, which is a common cause of headaches. By taking pantothenic acid, B-1 (thiamine), B-12 and B-6 (pyridoxine) vitamins, headaches can be prevented.

Beneficial Juices in Headache: Grapes, lemon, carrot, lettuce and spinach.

10 Things You Didn't Know About Wheatgrass

If anything ever screamed healthy, it's wheatgrass! The popularly-juiced, nutrient-rich grass is rich in chlorophyll, amino acids, vitamins, enzymes and supplements. But to many, wheatgrass remains something of an enigma. We dug deep to uncover some of the most interesting (we think!) facts about wheatgrass.

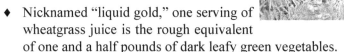

◆ Nicknamed "liquid gold," one serving of wheatgrass juice is the rough equivalent of one and a half pounds of dark leafy green vegetables.
◆ Because of its high chlorophyll content, wheatgrass has a strong alkalizing and detoxifying effect on the body.
◆ Growing wheatgrass at home is easy from seeds or whole grain wheat berries, by hand or with a sprouting kit. Perfect for having wheatgrass on hand for smoothies at all times!

- Like all chlorophyll-rich green plants, wheatgrass is high in oxygen and therefore an excellent source of natural energy.
- Wheatgrass is superior to other green plants because it has more than 100 elements needed by humans.
- Most often, wheatgrass is found as juice but powder supplements are also available and can be mixed into juices, smoothies or water. The best time-saving supplements are from freeze-dried organic wheatgrass juice powder
- Known to improve digestion, wheatgrass only takes one minute to digest.
- Even though the word "wheat" is in its name, wheatgrass is gluten-free.
- The best time to have wheatgrass juice is on an empty stomach and one hour before eating so that all the beneficial nutrients are completely available to the body for absorption.
- Depending on how toxic your body is, wheatgrass juice can cause headaches or increased bowel movements as the body detoxifies. Otherwise, expect lots of energy as the only side effect.

Chapter 20

Coronary Heart Disease

Coronary Heart Disease, chronic illness in which the coronary arteries, the vessels that supply oxygen-carrying blood to the heart, become narrowed and unable to carry a normal amount of blood. Most often, the coronary arteries become narrowed because of atherosclerosis, a process in which fatty deposits called plaque build up on the inside wall of an artery. Plaque is made of oily molecules known as cholesterol, fibrous proteins, calcium deposits, tiny blood cells known as platelets, and debris from dead cells. Plaque formation often begins in adolescence and progresses very slowly over the course of decades. Gradually, the growing plaque thickens the wall of the artery, reducing the space for blood to flow through.

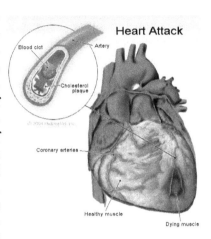

Heart Attack

When its blood supply is reduced, the heart does not receive sufficient oxygen. This oxygen deficit leads to two main consequences: chest pain known as angina pectoris, and heart attack, in which part of the heart dies because of oxygen deprivation. Coronary heart disease is the leading cause of death in the United States, responsible for about 515,000 deaths each year.

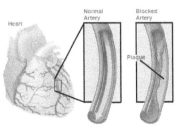

Angina Pectoris

A person who suffers from angina pectoris has coronary arteries that are wide enough to supply blood to the heart during normal activities, but too narrow to deliver sufficient blood and oxygen when extra work is required of the heart. An attack of angina develops when the heart must work harder than normal and the muscle cells that make up the heart do not receive enough oxygen.

Angina is typically felt as a heavy, squeezing pain in the centre of the chest. The pain may also spread to the neck, jaw, back, and left arm. An attack of angina may last for several minutes and is often brought on by physical activity, emotional stress, cold weather, or digestion of a heavy meal—all factors that can increase the heart's workload. Angina affects more than 6.6 million Americans.

Heart Attack

A heart attack, also known as a myocardial infarction, usually occurs when a blood clot forms inside a coronary artery at the site of an atherosclerotic plaque. The blood clot severely limits or completely cuts off blood flow to part of the heart. In a small percentage of cases, blood flow is cut off when the muscles in the artery wall contract suddenly, constricting the artery. This constriction, called vasospasm, can occur in an artery that is only slightly narrowed by atherosclerosis or even in a healthy artery.

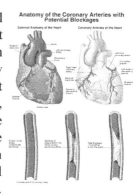

Anatomy of the Coronary Arteries with Potential Blockages

Regardless of the cause of a heart attack, the oxygen deprivation is so severe and prolonged that heart muscle cells begin to die for lack of oxygen. About 1.1 million people in the United States have a heart attack every year; the heart attacks prove fatal for about 40 percent of these people.

A person having a heart attack typically feels an intense, crushing pain in the chest, especially on the left side. The pain may radiate to the person's neck, jaw, and left arm. The pain is often similar to an attack of angina, but more intense and longer lasting. Other signs of a heart attack include profuse sweating, nausea, and vomiting. However, heart attack symptoms can vary greatly among people. In one study, about one-quarter of people who had a heart attack felt only mild symptoms and did not seek medical attention, and about 12 percent experienced no symptoms at all.

Some people have gradually worsening bouts of angina before having a heart attack. For others, a heart attack may be the first signal of heart trouble. No matter what a person's medical history, anyone who experiences symptoms of a heart attack should go to a hospital without delay. Oxygen deprivation can cause permanent damage to the heart within hours or even minutes, so the faster a heart attack patient receives treatment, the better the chance of survival.

Risk Factors

Some of the risk factors for coronary heart disease are beyond a person's control. For example, a person's risk of developing coronary heart disease increases with age. Hereditary factors may also increase the risk for the disease. Males were once thought to be at greater risk of coronary heart disease, but more recent studies show this is not true. About equal numbers of women and men develop coronary heart disease. Heart attacks in women are more likely to be fatal than in men. Women tend to develop the disease later in life than men do. This is because the sex hormone estrogen that circulates in women's bodies helps protect them against atherosclerosis. Therefore, most women do not develop coronary heart disease until after menopause, when levels of protective estrogen markedly decrease.

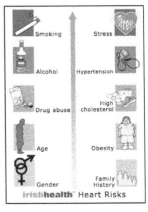

Other risk factors for coronary heart disease can be changed depending on a person's lifestyle. These modifiable risk factors include cigarette smoking, a sedentary lifestyle, obesity, diabetes mellitus, and hypertension (high blood pressure). Perhaps the most important modifiable risk factor, however, is high blood cholesterol. When excess cholesterol circulates in the blood, it deposits in the wall of the arteries, hastening the progression of atherosclerosis.

The amount of cholesterol in a person's bloodstream is partially determined by heredity, but it also depends on the amount of cholesterol and animal fat in the diet. In some parts of Asia and Africa where people consume very little fat and cholesterol, total blood cholesterol averages less than 150 milligrams per decilitre (mg/dl) and heart attacks are very rare. In the United States, where the typical diet includes many foods high in fat and cholesterol, total blood cholesterol averages about 200 mg/dl, and coronary heart disease is the leading cause of death.

Scientists have learned that cholesterol is especially dangerous when it is carried through the bloodstream as low-density lipoprotein (LDL), which is often known as "bad" cholesterol. By contrast, cholesterol in the form of high-density lipoprotein (HDL) actually lowers a person's risk of heart attack, and HDL is often referred to as "good" cholesterol.

Diagnosis

A variety of simple diagnostic methods may identify coronary heart disease before it becomes life threatening. Regular physical examinations, coupled with a person's family medical history, may alert a physician that a patient has a high risk for heart disease. Cholesterol screening, a blood test that measures cholesterol levels, can identify people at risk for atherosclerosis. In 2003 the United States Food and Drug Administration approved a new blood test that measures an enzyme called lipoprotein-associated phospholipase A2. Elevated levels of this enzyme indicate that a person is at increased risk for coronary heart disease. Studies have found that this blood test, known as the PLAC test, is a better indicator of coronary heart disease than cholesterol screening.

Chest pain, shortness of breath, and an abnormal pulse are some of the symptoms of coronary heart disease, but symptoms of heart disease may be different for every patient, and similar symptoms may also indicate a variety of other medical conditions. In a patient with chest pain, shortness of breath, or an abnormal pulse who also has risk factors for coronary heart disease, several types of tests help doctors make an accurate diagnosis.

An electrocardiogram (ECG, sometimes known as EKG) provides a graphical picture of the different phases of the heartbeat. An ECG recorded when a patient is at rest may indicate that the blood supply of the heart is not normal, and the ECG can often detect damage from a previous heart attack. In an exercise stress test, an ECG is recorded while a patient is performing physical activity such as walking on a treadmill or riding a stationary bicycle. As the intensity of exercise increases, the doctor looks for specific changes in the ECG that indicate the heart is not getting enough oxygen.

In cardiac catheterization, a long, thin, flexible tube called a catheter is threaded through an artery or vein to the patient's heart. Doctors collect information about the heart's function, such as pressure and blood flow in different chambers of the heart, by means of a device attached to the catheter. The catheter can also be used to perform coronary angiography, in which a dye that is visible on X rays is injected through the catheter into the coronary arteries. Moving and still X-ray pictures of the heart are taken, and the resulting images enable doctors to see where the coronary arteries are narrowed or obstructed by atherosclerosis.

Treatment

There is no cure for coronary heart disease. However, proper treatment can slow or even halt the progression of atherosclerosis so that the coronary arteries do not become further narrowed. Treatment can also help reduce the risk of a heart attack in people who have coronary heart disease.

The first step in fighting coronary heart disease is to make lifestyle changes to reduce risk factors. Doctors recommend that heart patients eat a low-fat diet and keep their blood cholesterol low. Most physicians believe LDL should be less than 100 mg/dl for patients with coronary heart disease. Patients are also encouraged to quit smoking, exercise regularly, and control high blood pressure and diabetes mellitus through diet or medication.

If a low-fat diet cannot reduce a person's cholesterol sufficiently, doctors may prescribe a cholesterol-lowering drug such as lovastatin, simvastatin, or pravastatin. Many different drugs are available to control angina. Nitroglycerin and similar drugs are the oldest such medications. More recently, two other types of drugs have become available, beta blockers and calcium channel blockers. All of these medications decrease the heart's oxygen demand (by slowing the heart rate or making the heart contract less vigorously), increase the heart's blood supply, or both. Sometimes patients may take a combination of these angina-relieving drugs. Finally, aspirin is sometimes recommended to help prevent a heart attack. Aspirin interferes with platelets, blood cells that are involved in blood clotting. In this way, the drug helps prevent the formation of a clot in a coronary artery.

Some patients may still suffer from angina even after making lifestyle changes and taking various medications. These patients may undergo coronary artery bypass surgery or percutaneous transluminal coronary angioplasty (PTCA) to help relieve their symptoms. In bypass surgery, a surgeon removes a length of blood vessel from elsewhere in the patient's body—usually a vein from the leg or an artery from the wrist. The surgeon then attaches one end of the blood vessel to the aorta and the other end to the coronary artery downstream of the blockage. Surgeons today commonly use an artery from the inside of the chest wall because bypasses made from this artery are very durable. The surgery creates a conduit for blood to flow through that bypasses the area narrowed by atherosclerosis. Sometimes multiple bypasses are created if more than one blockage exists. Bypass surgery became widely used in the early 1970s and is now performed on about 519,000 patients in the United States each year.

PTCA, often known as balloon angioplasty, is an alternative to bypass surgery, especially for patients with less extensive coronary artery disease. In this procedure, first performed in 1977, a catheter with a deflated balloon at its tip is threaded through the patient's arteries to the site of a blockage. The balloon is then inflated, crushing the atherosclerotic plaque and restoring normal flow of blood through the artery. Although balloon angioplasty is initially effective in most cases, a blockage may return after only a few months, resulting in a repeat artery narrowing known as restenosis. Cardiologists, physicians specializing in treating heart disorders, may use an expandable metal scaffolding called a stent to help prevent restenosis. The stent is placed in the artery at the time of angioplasty and helps keep the artery open. Nearly 600,000 balloon angioplasty procedures are performed in the United States each year.

When a person who may be having a heart attack arrives in the emergency room, doctors usually perform an ECG, which shows telltale changes when a heart attack is occurring. They may also order blood tests to detect the presence of chemicals released by injured heart muscle cells. The patient may be given drugs such as nitroglycerin and beta blockers, which decrease the heart's oxygen demand and help limit the amount of tissue damaged in the heart attack. Some patients are treated with a drug that dissolves blood clots, such as streptokinase or tissue-type plasminogen activator (t-PA). These drugs are most effective when given within an hour of the onset of chest pain. Other patients may have emergency balloon angioplasty or bypass surgery to restore blood flow to the heart muscle.

After a heart attack, a patient may remain in the hospital for several days. At first, he or she may stay in a coronary care unit (CCU), an intensive care unit designed specifically for heart attack patients. In the CCU, the patient is monitored constantly with an ECG, and specially trained doctors and nurses are on hand to treat abnormal heart rhythms or other complications that may develop. Before the patient leaves the hospital, doctors may order an exercise stress test, coronary angiography, or other tests to evaluate whether the person should have angioplasty or bypass surgery.

Natural Treatment for Coronary Heart Disease

Apples contain heart stimulating properties and help strengthen the heart muscles. Eating an apple every morning for breakfast helps combat coronary heart disease. You can also extract 1 glass fresh apple juice and take it daily on an empty stomach.

Grapes are known to reduce heart palpitation and chest pain. It is recommended to take an all grape diet for a few days to help control coronary heart disease. Drinking a glass of fresh grape juice also helps prevent heart attack.

Amla or Indian Gooseberry tones the heart functions and strengthens the immune system. It is recommended to take Amla juice on a daily basis to treat Coronary heart disease.

Terminalia Arjuna is a herbal cure for combating heart disease effectively. It relieves mental stress, decreases LDL cholesterol and is a potent cardioprotective agent. It is recommended to take Terminalia Arjuna dietary supplements on a daily basis for dealing with this condition.

Onions are also highly beneficial for combating heart disease. They lower the level of cholesterol and improve the functioning of the heart. Take 1 tsp of raw onion juice on an empty stomach every morning for best results.

Vitamin E improves the functioning of the heart and enhances circulation. Green leafy vegetables and outer leaves of cabbage are recommended to treat heart disease.

Beneficial Juices in Coronary Heart Disease: Red grapes, lemon, cucumber, carrot, Amla, beet and spinach.

Drinking Fruit Juice Regularly Can Help You Prevent Heart Disease

Heart disease is a general term used for diseases that interfere with the vascular system, or more precisely attack the heart and veins, such as coronary heart disease, heart attack, high blood pressure and chest pain (angina).

No one wants suffering from heart disease. Therefore, we need to know what causes it and how to prevent it. Many factors cause a person vulnerable to heart disease. All we know so far, heart disease due to age or heredity.

The main factor causing a person vulnerable to heart disease are lifestyle issues. Thus, heart disease can be prevented by adopting a healthy lifestyle.

Many vegetables that can be used for juice therapy, such as spinach, celery, carrots, tomatoes, squash, asparagus, corn, kale, and broccoli. All types of nuts can also, such as soybeans, green beans, green beans, sweet peas, and peppers.

While fruit juice can be used for therapy, such as mango, pear, avocado, watermelon, grapes, star fruit, pineapple, passion fruit , rambutan, melon, litchi, and olives. Below is one example that could juice your own potion at home.

Melon Longan Juice (for 1 cup)

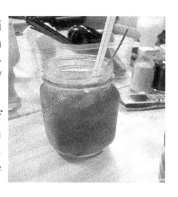

Ingredients: 100 grams of melon, litchi cut into pieces 100 g, chopped 60 g green beans, cut into pieces 60 ml water 1 tablespoon honey 1 tablespoon lemon juice/ juice 3 pieces ice cubes.

Directions: Enter the pieces of melon, litchi, green beans, water, lemon juice, and ice cubes to the blender jar. Puree until smooth then strain. Pour the juice into a glass and drink immediately.

Strawberry Juice Combination (for 1 cup)

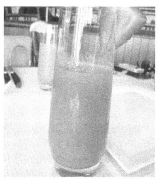

Ingredients: 100 grams of strawberries, cut into pieces 100 grams of tomatoes, chopped 60 ml of fresh non-fat milk 1 tablespoon honey 1 tablespoon lime juice / lemon 3 ice cubes

Directions: Enter chunks strawberries, tomatoes, fresh liquid milk, lemon juice and chunks of ice cubes into the blender. Puree until soft portion and serve immediately.

Chapter 21

Influenza

Influenza, also known as flu, contagious infection primarily of the respiratory tract. Influenza is sometimes referred to as grippe. Influenza is caused by a virus transmitted from one person to another in droplets coughed or sneezed into the air. It is characterized by coldlike symptoms plus chills, fever, headaches, muscle aches, and fatigue. Most people recover completely in about a week. But some people are vulnerable to complications such as bronchitis and pneumonia. This group includes children with asthma, people with heart or lung disease, and the elderly. In the United States, people age 65 and older account for about 90 percent of influenza-associated deaths.

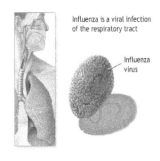

Influenza is a viral infection of the respiratory tract

Influenza virus

In addition to humans, influenza occurs in pigs, horses, and several other mammals as well as in certain wild and domesticated birds. At least some influenza viruses can jump from one species to another. For example, in late 1997 a strain of the influenza virus in chickens began to infect humans in Hong Kong, leading to a massive effort to eradicate the strain.

Because influenza is highly contagious and spreads easily, it usually appears as epidemics—that is, outbreaks involving many people. If an outbreak spreads around the world—not uncommon in this age of rapid international travel—it is called a pandemic.

Many millions of people develop the flu each year. In most years less than 1 percent of those infected die. Nonetheless, this translates into large numbers. The United States Centres for Disease Control and Prevention (CDC) estimates that influenza causes more than 20,000 deaths in the United States each year; combined, influenza and pneumonia are among the nation's ten leading causes of death. During epidemics and pandemics, death rates soar. The influenza pandemic that occurred from 1918 to 1919—the worst on record—killed about 500,000 people in the United States and from 20 million to 50 million people worldwide.

Cause

The word *influenza* is derived from the Latin word *influentia.* Italians in the early 16th century first applied the word influenza to outbreaks of any epidemic disease because they blamed such outbreaks on the influence of heavenly bodies. The first known use of the name specifically for the flu occurred in 1743 when an epidemic swept through Rome and its environs.

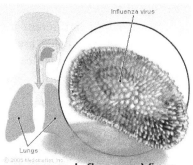

Influenza Virus

Today scientists know that members of the family Orthomyxoviridae, a group of viruses that infect vertebrate animals, cause influenza. The virus consists of an inner core of the genetic material ribonucleic acid (RNA) surrounded by a protein coat and an outer lipid (fatty) envelope. From this envelope, spikes of proteins called hemagglutinin and neuraminidase stick out. Hemagglutinin enables the virus to bind to and invade cells, and neuraminidase allows the virus to move among cells. But these proteins also act as antigens—that is, they are recognized as foreign matter by the human or other host organism, and this recognition triggers an immune response in the host.

There are three types of influenza viruses, known as A, B, and C. Type A, the most dangerous, infects a wide variety of mammals and birds. It causes the most cases of the disease in humans and is the type most likely to become epidemic. Type B infects humans and birds, producing a milder disease that can also cause epidemics. Type C apparently infects only humans. It typically produces either a very mild illness indistinguishable from a common cold or no symptoms at all. Type C does not cause epidemics.

Influenza type A and B viruses continually change. Some changes involve a series of genetic mutations that, over a period of time, cause a gradual evolution of the virus. Called antigenic drift, this process accounts for most of the changes in influenza viruses that occur from one year to the next. Other changes, less common but more injurious, involve abrupt changes in the hemagglutinin or neuraminidase. This type of change is called antigenic shift and results in a new subtype of the virus. Type A viruses undergo both kinds of transformations;

influenza type B viruses apparently change only by the process of antigenic drift.

Scientists further differentiate virus subtypes into strains, generally named for the geographic area where they were first detected. For example, the strains that caused the most infections during the 2001-2002 flu season in the Northern Hemisphere were type A New Caledonia and Moscow strains and Type B Sichuan strain.

Once a person has been infected by a specific strain of influenza, he or she has built up immunity to that strain in the form of antibodies. The person's immune system then can recognize the strain's hemagglutinin or neuraminidase and attack them if they reappear. The antibodies offer some protection against antigenic drifts, but not against antigenic shifts. Thus, because the viruses continually change, they can cause repeated waves of infection, even among people previously infected.

Scientists do not understand exactly what causes antigenic shifts. One leading theory suggests that a human strain and an animal strain recombine to create a new strain. This strain has the ability to infect humans but has antigens on its surface that are unfamiliar to the human immune system.

Transmission

Influenza viruses pass from person to person mainly in droplets expelled during sneezes and coughs. When a person breathes in virus-laden droplets, the hemagglutinin on the surface of the virus binds to enzymes in the mucous membranes that line the respiratory tract. The enzymes, known as proteases, 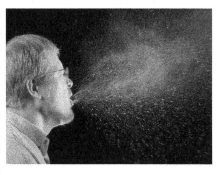 cut the hemagglutinin in two, which enables the virus to gain entry into cells and begin to multiply. These proteases are common in the respiratory and digestive tracts but not elsewhere, which is why the flu causes primarily a respiratory illness with occasional gastrointestinal symptoms. In the 1990s scientists discovered that some flu strains also can use the enzyme plasmin to cut hemagglutinin. Plasmin is common throughout the body, enabling the flu strains to infect a variety of tissues.

Although an influenza epidemic can occur at any time of year, flu season in temperate regions typically begins with the approach of winter—November in the Northern Hemisphere, April in the Southern Hemisphere. Flu viruses spread more easily during cold weather because people tend to spend more time crowded together in homes and schools, as well as buses, subways, and other places with poor ventilation. An epidemic may be restricted to a town or city or may quickly spread geographically as infected people travel aboard motor vehicles, airplanes, and ships.

Symptoms and Diagnosis

Influenza is an acute disease with a rapid onset and pronounced symptoms. After the influenza virus invades a person's body, an incubation period of one to two days passes before symptoms appear. Classic symptoms include sore throat, dry cough, stuffed or runny nose, chills, fever with temperatures as high as 39° C (103° F), aching muscles and joints, headache, loss of appetite, occasional nausea and

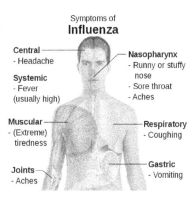

Symptoms of
Influenza

Central
- Headache

Systemic
- Fever
(usually high)

Muscular
- (Extreme) tiredness

Joints
- Aches

Nasopharynx
- Runny or stuffy nose
- Sore throat
- Aches

Respiratory
- Coughing

Gastric
- Vomiting

vomiting, and fatigue. For most people flu symptoms begin to subside after two to three days and disappear in seven to ten days. However, coughing and fatigue may persist for two or more weeks.

Death from influenza itself is rare. But influenza can aggravate underlying medical conditions, such as heart or lung disease. Invading influenza viruses produce inflammation in the lining of the respiratory tract, damage that increases the risk that secondary infections will develop. Common complications include bronchitis, sinusitis, and bacterial pneumonia, occurring most frequently in the elderly, people on chemotherapy, and people with acquired immunodeficiency syndrome (AIDS) or other diseases that compromise the immune system. If properly treated, these complications seldom are fatal.

Because influenza is so common and exhibits standard symptoms, doctors often diagnose the illness based on the season and whether flu cases have recently been reported in the area. To prove a diagnosis of influenza in a patient, the virus must be isolated from the person's nasal or cough secretions or blood and identified under a microscope.

Treatment and Prevention

There is no specific cure for influenza. Recommended treatment usually consists of bed rest and increased intake of nonalcoholic fluids until fever and other symptoms lessen in severity. Certain drugs have been found effective in lessening flu symptoms, but medical efforts against the disease focus chiefly on prevention by means of vaccines that create immunity.

Drugs That Ease Symptoms

No drugs can cure influenza, but certain antiviral medicines can relieve flu symptoms. Available by prescription, these drugs provide modest relief, but only if taken on the first or second day of symptoms. The drugs amantadine (sold under the brand name *Symmetrel*) and rimantadine *(Flumadine),* both in pill form, work against hemagglutinin and are effective in treating type A influenza. Two other drugs inhibit neuraminidase and are effective against both type A and type B strains: oseltamivir *(Tamiflu)* is in pill form and zanamivir *(Relenza)* is an inhalant.

Vaccines

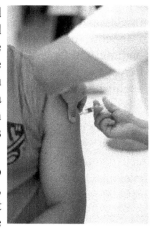

A flu vaccine consists of greatly weakened or killed flu viruses, or fragments of dead viruses. Antigens in the vaccine stimulate a person's immune system to produce antibodies against the viruses. If the flu viruses invade a vaccinated person at a later time, the sensitized immune system recognizes the antigens and quickly responds to help destroy the viruses.

About 5 to 10 percent of people who receive a flu vaccine experience mild, temporary side effects, typically soreness at the injection site. Young children who have not previously been exposed to the influenza virus are most likely to have side effects.

Flu viruses constantly change so different virus strains must be incorporated in vaccines from one year to the next. Scientists try to provide a good match between the vaccine and the most serious virus strains circulating at the time. But because it takes months to manufacture and distribute vaccines, decisions on their composition must be made well before the start of each flu season. Each February experts at the World Health Organization (WHO) recommend the composition of the vaccine for the forthcoming winter in the Northern Hemisphere; a second recommendation is made in September for vaccines to be used in the Southern Hemisphere. Typically vaccines contain antigens from three virus strains, usually two type A and one type B.

According to the CDC, the success of flu vaccines varies from one person to another. In healthy young adults, the vaccines are 70 to 90 percent effective in preventing the disease. In the elderly and people with certain chronic medical conditions, the vaccines are less effective in preventing illness but help reduce the severity of an infection and the risk of major complications or death. Studies show that flu vaccines reduce hospitalization by about 70 percent and death by about 85 percent among elderly people.

Recommendations for Flu Shots

The CDC recommends annual flu shots for people who are at high risk for developing serious complications as a result of an influenza infection. This group includes all people age 65 and older; people in nursing homes and other facilities that house people with chronic medical conditions; people with chronic heart, lung or kidney disease, diabetes, an impaired immune system, or severe forms of anemia; children and adolescents with conditions treated for long periods of time with aspirin (which makes them vulnerable to Reye's syndrome); and women who will be in the second or third trimester of pregnancy during the influenza season.

To help stop the disease's spread, the CDC also recommends vaccination for health-care workers, employees of nursing homes and chronic-care facilities, and household members of people in high-risk groups. Doctors encourage individuals who travel to areas of the world where influenza viruses circulate to receive the most current vaccine, particularly if they are at higher risk of complications.

It takes the human immune system one to two weeks after vaccination to develop antibodies to the flu antigens. According to the CDC, the best time to get flu shots in the United States is between October 1 and mid-November—sufficiently in advance of the peak of influenza activity, which in the United States generally lasts from late December until early March.

Flu shots must be given annually for two reasons. First, antibody protection provided by the vaccine decreases during the year following vaccination. Second, vaccines created for pre-existing viral strains may not work against new strains; nor does an infection with one flu strain confer immunity to infection by another strain.

Home Remedies for Influenza

Turmeric: In one cup of warm milk add about one teaspoon of turmeric powder and drink it three times in a day. This remedy is very useful to treat influenza and you can safely try this remedy on your kids too, if they are suffering form influenza.

Onion Juice: It is also beneficial to take onion juice and honey in equal quantities for about one week in the treatment of influenza. Onion juice has medicinal properties and helps the body to fight against the influenza viruses.

Holy Basil Leaves: Keep half litre water for boiling in a vessel. Add fresh holy basil leaves and slices of ginger into this boiling water and keep on boiling. After some time put off the gas and allow it to cool. Strain it and drink this medicinal tea, which will give quick relief form cold, cough and runny nose. This is one of the most recommended home remedies for influenza.

Ginger Juice: Take half teaspoon of ginger juice and add two teaspoon of honey and half teaspoon of pepper powder. Mix all these ingredients well and have it three times in a day. This remedy is very beneficial if started at the onset of influenza.

Diet: Reduce the intake of solid food; instead go for fruit juices and vegetable juices. This will help the immunity system to work well. Avoid too much spicy food and avoid cheese, rice and white flour. Eat warm food and avoid eating stale food or outside food. Avoid red meat and stay away form smoking, alcohol and tobacco.

Drink Boiled Water: Avoid drinking outside outer. If you have to go out of the house for some work, then carry your home water with you in one bottle. At home also drink only boiled water. This will give fast relief form influenza.

Avoid Having Bath: Influenza symptoms can become worse if you will take bath. Hence with cold water sponge your body instead of taking regular bath. You can skip taking bath for two to three days. In case your kid has got influenza, then follow this without fail. Or else their cold, cough and runny nose problems will not get cured.

Beneficial Juices in Influenza: Apricot, orange, lemon, grapefruit, pineapple, carrot, onion and spinach.

Horseradish and lemon juice: the potent ethers in fresh grated horseradish dissolve mucus in the sinuses and bronchial tubes quickly and effectively; mixing it with fresh lemon juice doubles its efficacy; grate fresh horseradish into a bowel, add enough fresh lemon juice to make a paste, take 1/2 tsp 2-3 times a day, as needed.

Carrot, celery, parsley, spinach juice: this blend is super-rich in potassium, which quickly reduces acidity throughout the system, thereby commencing the detoxification process required for complete cure and recovery.

This blend also contains the full range of organic minerals and other nutrients required to sustain convalescing patients, without stuffing them full of solid foods; 8 oz/4 oz/2 oz/4 oz, 1-2 pints daily, taken in small doses throughout the day.

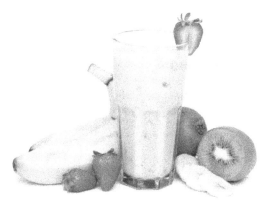

Other beneficial foods: lettuce juice; carrot and radish juice; whole lemon puree; grapefruit juice (in distilled warm water); distilled warm water.

Foods to avoid: all cooked and solid foods; pasteurized milk; coffee, tea; sweet soft drinks.

Chapter 22

Insomnia

Insomnia or sleeplessness is a modern age complaint which is becoming more common due to worry, mental strain, over-use of stimulants like tea and coffee, lack of physical exercise, sleeping in over-crowded and ill-ventilated rooms, etc. Occasional sleeplessness is but natural, but persistent insomnia is a disease that should be treated because it can greatly affect the overall health of person.

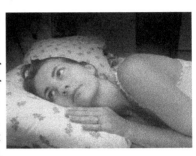

Symptoms of Insomnia
♦ Heaviness in head
♦ Feeling of pain in head
♦ Nausea
♦ Feeling of tiredness and weakness
♦ Body ache
♦ Burning sensation in eyes
♦ Irritation

Causes of Insomnia

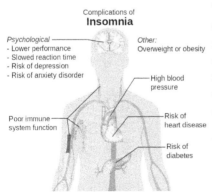

Complications of
Insomnia

Psychological
- Lower performance
- Slowed reaction time
- Risk of depression
- Risk of anxiety disorder

Other:
Overweight or obesity

High blood
pressure

Poor immune
system function

Risk of
heart disease

Risk of
diabetes

The main causes of Insomnia are digestive disorder, Constipation, mental tension, fear and worry etc. Even addiction to T.V. and reading of books, use of Tea, Coffee and other intoxicants also delay the sleep. By in ordinate increase in blood flow toward head the sleep disappears. Mind obsessed by thoughts at the time of sleep, becomes tense and disturbed and vanishes the sleep. Obscene literature disturbs the mind and prevents sleep.

Treatment of Insomnia by Nature Cure

Water Treatment

For immediate relief, Natural bath or hot footbath is useful. Spinal pack also promotes sleep. In case of application of Chest pack enhances sleep Insomnia due to breathing disorder. In winter season bathing with water of neutral temperature before sleep is beneficial. After that Cold mudpack may be applied over abdomen and forehead. Regular use of Cold hipbath is also beneficial.

For getting permanent relief from this disease cleansing of bowel by taking lemon water enema is also beneficial. Such patients should give up intoxicants like tea, coffee etc. to get quick benefit. The bedroom for such patients should also be sufficiently airy and open.

Beneficial Juices in Insomnia: Apple, grapes, lemon, lettuce, carrot and celery.

Cherry Juice Beneficial in Curing Insomnia

The modern lifestyles have caused an increased number of problems and insomnia is one of them. Experts have disclosed that one in three adults is suffering from this problem.

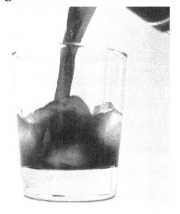

A recent study reveals that cherry juice is beneficial in curing insomnia. The study was headed by Wilfred Pigeon, who is a Psychiatrist from the University of Rochester in New York.

The researchers have discovered that after consuming a glass of unsweetened cherry juice, two times a day; the respondents had a sound sleep at night, as compared to those people, who drank the similar quantity of any other juice.

Mr. Pigeon has revealed that the reason behind it is that melatonin is present in a large amount in this fruit. Melatonin is a hormone, which controls the body's clock.

In the study the sleeping patterns of respondents were monitored for two routines. In the first routine, they consumed cherry juice while in the second, they consumed some other juice.

The scientists concluded that cherry juice was beneficial in increasing 17 minutes of sleep.

Mr. Pigeon said that many of the medicines used for treating insomnia have some or the other side effects, therefore, this is a better option for such people.

Cherry juice is also used to treat the pain, which is caused by arthritis as it contains, anthocyanins that is a compound responsible for alleviating inflammation in the body.

Chapter 23

Jaundice

Jaundice or Icterus, yellowing of the skin, conjunctivae, and mucous membranes caused by excessive amounts of bile pigments in blood tissues. These pigments, normally present in blood as a result of the breakdown of hemoglobin in red blood cells, are filtered through the liver and excreted in feces. Excessive amounts of these pigments produce four types of jaundice.

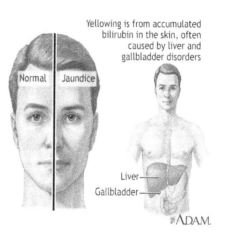

Yellowing is from accumulated bilirubin in the skin, often caused by liver and gallbladder disorders

Normal Jaundice

Liver—
Gallbladder—

✴A.D.A.M.

In hemolytic jaundice there is increased production of bile pigment because of red blood-cell damage. This damage can be caused by antibodies created by a mismatched blood transfusion. In infants the antibodies can be caused by prenatal mismatch between the Rh factor in the infant's blood and that of the mother.

Newborns can also be jaundiced as a consequence of the condition known as hyperbilirubinemia. In these cases, there is a temporary defect in synthesis of the enzyme that breaks down bile to an excretable form.

Hepatocellular jaundice occurs when liver cells are damaged either by viruses, or by excessive intake of alcohol, and lose the ability to process pigment.

Obstructive jaundice follows physical obstruction of the ducts that transport pigment from the liver to the intestine. Blockage can be due to gallstones, tumor, or inflammation.

Beneficial Juices in Jaundice: Lemon, grapes, pear, carrot, celery, spinach, beet and cucumber.

Jaundice | 131

Juice Remedies for Jaundice

Make a mixture of a glass of fresh tomato juice, a pinch of salt, pepper and taken to patient early in the morning. Make a mixture of 1 glass of sugarcane juice and juice of half a lime, taken this juice 2 times everyday. Take leaves of snake gourd, 15 gram of dry leaves and 250 ml of water, make a mixture from this and then boiling it, after taken this are a one time in a day.

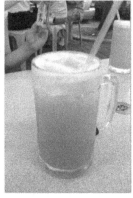

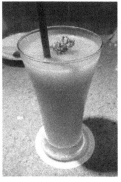

Take a carrot juice and drink it regularly after meals at least for a month. You can take a powder as well as juice for Indian drug Amlaki or Indian gooseberry. Take a grinding of bitter gourd and water; make a mixture from this and given this mixture to a patient two times in a day. Make a mixture of 1 tbs. of honey and smash 1 matured banana, after eat this mixture 2 times in a day.

Chapter 24

Kidney Disorders

The kidneys are two bean-shaped organs, about 5 inches long and 3 inches wide. They are dark red in colour, and located on either side of your spine in the middle of your back, just below your rib cage. The right kidney lies a little lower than the left kidney. The kidneys together with the bladder, two ureters and single urethra constitute the urinary system.

Anatomy of the Kidney

Calyces

Renal Pelvis

Renal Artery

Medulla

Renal Vein

Ureter

Cortex

Each kidney is covered with a transparent, fibrous membrane called a renal capsule which protects it against infection and trauma. Each kidney contains millions of microscopically thin structures called nephrons which filters the blood and causes waste to be eliminated in the form of urine. The kidneys do not weigh much - approximately 0.5 percent of your body weight.

Too many waste products that build up in the bloodstream can cause a wide range of kidney disorders may develop. Diabetes and high blood pressure are the major causes of kidney disease. By managing your sugar levels, checking your blood pressure regularly, having regular blood and urine tests to monitor kidney health and function will help to ward off kidney disease. In addition, eat healthy, balanced meals, exercise regularly and stop smoking are a few small changes that can make a huge difference to your kidney function.

Function of the Kidneys

The kidneys have several important functions and they include:

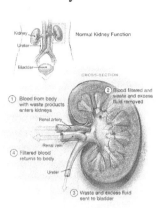

- ◆ Separates urea, mineral salts, toxins and other waste products from the blood
- ◆ Conserves water, salts and electrolytes
- ◆ Filters metabolic wastes from the blood plasma and excretes it from the body
- ◆ Removes and breaks down toxins in the body by getting rid of it in the urine
- ◆ Balances the volume of body fluid and mineral content
- ◆ Responsible for ensuring that blood pressure remains steady over the long term
- ◆ Balances the volume of body fluid and mineral content
- ◆ Responsible for ensuring that blood pressure remains steady over the long term
- ◆ Excretes extra acid that the body produces
- ◆ Excretes water and electrolytes to match water intake and endogenous production
- ◆ Secretes hormones Erythropoietin (EPO) to make more red blood cells
- ◆ Activates Vitamin D to maintain healthy bones

Diagnosing Kidney Disease

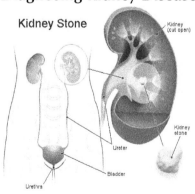

- ◆ Polycystic kidney disease (PKD) is an inherited disease in which numerous cysts filled with fluid form in the kidneys, causing them to become enlarged.
- ◆ Nephrotic syndrome is a kidney disease characterized by a massive leak of protein (albumin) into the urine (proteinuria), a low blood level of albumin due to the large amounts lost in the urine, an increased level of cholesterol

in the blood and retention of fluid in the body (edema) causing swelling.

- ♦ Lupus nephritis is an inflammation of the kidney caused by a disease of the immune system, systemic lupus erythematosus (SLE).
- ♦ Diabetic nephropathy is a kidney condition that occurs as a result of diabetes.
- ♦ Glomerulonephritis is a type of kidney disease caused by inflammation of the internal kidney structures.
- ♦ Pyelonephritis is an infection of the kidney and the ureters.
- ♦ Rhabdomyolysis is a disorder involving injury to the kidney.
- ♦ Kidney stone is a hard, stone-like mass developed from crystals that forms in the kidneys or urinary tract
- ♦ Renal tubular acidosis (RTA) occurs when the kidneys fail to excrete acids into the urine, and as a result a person's blood remains too acidic.
- ♦ Acute renal failure occurs when your kidneys stop working
- ♦ Chronic renal failure is a condition in which kidney function gradually declines

Help for Kidney Diseases

Treating kidney disease and conditions generally depends on the type of condition that the individual may have. Medications include several prescription drugs such as antibiotics and steroids. People suffering from high blood pressure and diabetes should monitor and control these conditions to prevent further damage to their kidneys. If kidney failure occurs, dialysis which involves the blood being filtered by an artificial kidney machine is required. In cases where kidney failure is severe and irreversible, a kidney transplant may be necessary.

Natural herbal remedies are often used in combination with synthetic drugs to treat kidney problems. Not only are these herbs gentle to use on the body but they provide the same benefits without harsh side effects.

Herbs such as Agathosma betulina (Buchu) possess diuretic prop-erties and acts as urinary antiseptic while Berberis vulgaris (Barberry) improves immune functioning and is excellent for kidney stones, gall-bladder problems and an enlarged spleen. Other herbal ingredients that are extremely beneficial for kidney health include Polygonum multiflo-rum, Schizandra chinensis and Trigonella foenum-graecum.

Beneficial Juices in Kidney Disorders: Apple, orange, lemon, cucumber, cucumber, carrot, celery, parsley and beet.

Pomegranate Juice Beneficial For Kidney Disease Patients

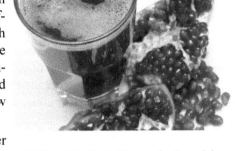

Pomegranate juice, which is rich in antioxidants, offers a wide variety of health benefits to kidney disease patients including managing blood pressure and lowering cholesterol, a new study has claimed.

Lilach Shema and her colleagues from the Western Galilee Medical Centre in Israel investigated the long-term effects of drinking pomegranate juice on heart disease risk factors like high cholesterol and blood pressure in kidney disease patients.

They randomised 101 dialysis patients to receive about three-and-a-half ounces of pomegranate juice or placebo, three times a week.

After one year, the number of blood pressure drugs patients took decreased in 22 percent of patients drinking pomegranate juice compared to 7.7 percent in the placebo group, while an increase was documented in 12.2 percent of patients drinking pomegranate juice compared to 34.6 percent in the placebo group.

They also found that patients who drank pomegranate juice had healthier blood pressure and cholesterol levels and less plaque build-up in their arteries.

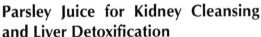

Parsley Juice for Kidney Cleansing and Liver Detoxification

Parsley juice is a potent and concentrated version of all the nutrition in the herb, including a rich array of vitamins, minerals, antioxidants, enzymes, chlorophyll and volatile oils. Parsley is also known to be especially good for kidney cleansing and liver detoxification and in this we will suggest two recipes for this purpose, the first using a juicer and the second a blender.

Importantly, parsley should not be used in large amounts by pregnant women or those taking blood thinning medication. There is also conflicting advice regarding using it for people suffering from kidney disease. Some medical resources caution against using too much parsley as it contains substances known as oxalates, sometimes suggested to be avoided by people with kidney problems.

On the other hand, parsley has a long history as a beneficial herb for the kidneys and both the fresh plant and dried tea are often recommended for kidney infections or to help dissolve kidney stones.

Additionally, parsley, like most green superfoods, is generally considered too powerful to drink on its own and is better mixed with other complementary fruits and vegetables. Some of the best of these for kidney cleansing and liver detoxification include:

Watermelon
Watermelon is great for flushing the kidneys and watermelon seeds are said to be especially beneficial for kidney stones. If this is something you're concerned with, then look for a watermelon with the brown seeds rather than the seedless varieties.

Celery
Celery strengthens the liver and kidneys and helps to eliminate toxins. Unfortunately conventionally grown celery often has a high pesticide load so organic is definitely preferable.

Beetroot
Beetroot is an excellent cleanser and detoxifier, particularly for the liver. It is also said to purify the blood and help eliminate calcium oxalate stones.

Carrot
Carrot juice is another powerful body cleanser and particularly good for the kidneys. Unfortunately carrots can absorb pesticides and heavy metals from the ground they're grown in so must be organic.

Cucumber
Cucumber is a diuretic that can help flush uric acid out of the body and dissolve kidney stones. The skin is full of antioxidants but conventionally grown cucumbers have a significant pesticide load and

are also usually coated with wax. If you can't find organic cucumbers you'd be better off peeling them.

Lemon Juice
Lemon juice from a fresh lemon is an excellent cleanser and can help dissolve mineral deposits that lead to calcium oxalate stones. Lemon will also help delay oxidization of the other juices.

The two recipes below use different combinations of these ingredients for the juicer and the blender. Feel free to mix it up depending on what you have available. Or, for the ultimate superfood kidney cleanser and liver detox, first juice and then blend and combine all the ingredients together.

Parsley Juice with a Juicer
While you could use as standard centrifugal juicer, unless it's a particularly good one you often won't get much out of even a whole bunch of parsley. In the past I've tried squeezing the parsley heads into a ball between two loads of carrots, but in the end I realized a proper masticating juicer just makes more sense.

While they cost more initially, a masticating juicer is an essential item if you want to juice green superfoods like parsley, spinach or wheatgrass effectively. They also get far more out of regular fruit and veggies as well as keeping the heat and oxidization right down. This greatly improves both the quantity and quality of the juice they deliver.

Carrot, Celery, Beetroot, Cucumber, Lemon and Parsley Juice

Ingredients
+ Two large or three medium organic carrots.
+ Two sticks of organic celery.
+ One medium beetroot.
+ One small or half a large organic cucumber with the peel (peel non-organic cucumbers).
+ The juice of one large or two small lemons (always discard citrus seeds).
+ One ounce of organic parsley soaked in warm water (roughly half an average sized bunch).

Method
Pour lemon juice into your collection container along with a couple of

ice cubes. This will help lessen the degradation of the juice.

Push all of the ingredients through the juicer, alternating between the harder carrots and beetroot with the softer cucumber and celery. Scrunch the parsley up into a ball and feed it through between the harder vegetables. Once again, you will get much more parsley juice out of a masticating juicer than a centrifugal one.

Stir to mix the juice and drink immediately.

Parsley Juice in a Blender
A well-designed blender can blend up parsley heads into a refreshing smoothie, where you're getting all of the health benefits of parsley in an easily digestible form.

Cheap ones may struggle to chop it up, but a powerful blender will turn parsley into an extremely healthy, bright green puree.

Watermelon, Cucumber, Lemon and Parsley Smoothie
While you could chop up watermelon and juice it, it's so high in water content that it is especially suitable for blending. The same goes for cucumber.

There are also beneficial nutrients in the seeds of both watermelon and cucumber, so if you're not afraid of a little texture, then keep the seeds in (the better the blender the smaller these will be chopped up).

Ingredients
♦ Half an ounce of organic parsley (less is needed than in juicing as the whole herb is used).
♦ The juice of one large or two small lemons (minus the seeds).
♦ One large organic cucumber, diced with the peel on and seeds kept (peel first if you can't find organic).
♦ As much watermelon with the seeds as you can fit into the blender.

Method
Blend all these ingredients up until you can see the parsley leaves finely blended and the watermelon seeds chopped up into small pieces. Drink immediately.

This smoothie is extremely refreshing and very good for cleaning the kidneys. Remember though that watermelon really doesn't keep once blended so you'd want to drink this smoothie right away.

Chapter 25
Liver Ailments

Liver, largest internal organ of the human body. The liver, which is part of the digestive system, performs more than 500 different functions, all of which are essential to life. Its essential functions include helping the body to digest fats, storing reserves of nutrients, filtering poisons and wastes from the blood, synthesizing a variety of proteins, and regulating the levels of many chemicals found in the bloodstream. The liver is unique among the body's vital organs in that it can regenerate,

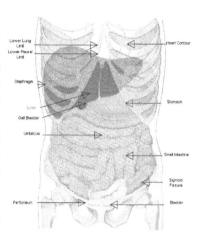

or grow back, cells that have been destroyed by some short-term injury or disease. But if the liver is damaged repeatedly over a long period of time, it may undergo irreversible changes that permanently interfere with function.

Structure of the Liver

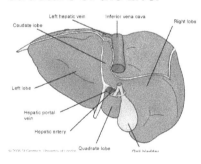

The human liver is a dark red-brown organ with a soft, spongy texture. It is located at the top of the abdomen, on the right side of the body just below the diaphragm—a sheet of muscle tissue that separates the lungs from the abdominal organs. The lower part of the rib cage covers the liver, protecting it from injury. In a healthy adult, the liver weighs about 1.5 kg (3 lb) and is about 15 cm (6 in) thick.

Despite its many complex functions, the liver is relatively simple in structure. It consists of two main lobes, left and right, which overlap slightly. The right lobe has two smaller lobes attached to it, called the quadrate and caudate lobes.

Each lobe contains many thousands of units called lobules that are the building blocks of the liver. Lobules are six-sided structures each about 1 mm (0.04 in) across. A tiny vein runs through the centre of each lobule and eventually drains into the hepatic vein, which carries blood out of the liver. Hundreds of cubed-shaped liver cells, called hepatocytes, are arranged around the lobule's central vein in a radiating pattern. On the outside surface of each lobule are small veins, ducts, and arteries that carry fluids to and from the lobules. As the liver does its work, nutrients are collected, wastes are removed, and chemical substances are released into the body through these vessels.

Unlike most organs, which have a single blood supply, the liver receives blood from two sources. The hepatic artery delivers oxygen-rich blood from the heart, supplying about 25 percent of the liver's blood. The liver also receives oxygen-depleted blood from the hepatic portal vein. This vein, which is the source of 75 percent of the liver's blood supply, carries blood to the liver that has traveled from the digestive tract, where it collects nutrients as food is digested. These nutrients are delivered to the liver for further processing or storage.

Tiny blood vessel branches of the hepatic artery and the hepatic portal vein are found around each liver lobule. This network of blood vessels is responsible for the vast amount of blood that flows through the liver—about 1.4 litres (about 3 pt) every minute. Blood exits the liver through the hepatic vein, which eventually drains into the heart.

Functions of the Liver

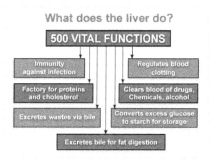

One of the liver's primary jobs is to store energy in the form of glycogen, which is made from a type of sugar called glucose. The liver removes glucose from the blood when blood glucose levels are high. Through a process called glycogenesis, the liver combines the glucose molecules in long chains to create glycogen, a carbohydrate that provides a stored form of energy. When the amount of glucose in the blood falls below the level required to meet the body's needs, the liver reverses this reaction, transforming glycogen into glucose.

Another crucial function of the liver is the production of bile, a yellowish-brown liquid containing salts necessary for the digestion of lipids, or fats. These salts are produced within the lobules. Bile leaves the liver through a network of ducts and is transported to the gallbladder, which concentrates the bile and releases it into the small intestine.

Vitamins are also stored in the liver. Drawing on the nutrient-rich blood in the hepatic portal vein, the liver collects and stores supplies of vitamins A, D, E, and K. The B vitamins are also stored here, including a two- to four-year supply of Vitamin B_{12}.

The liver also functions as the body's chemical factory. Several important proteins found in the blood are produced in the liver. One of these proteins, albumin, helps retain calcium and other important substances in the bloodstream. Albumin also helps regulate the movement of water from the bloodstream into the body's tissues. The liver also produces globin, one of the two components that form hemoglobin—the oxygen-carrying substance in red blood cells. Certain globulins, a group of proteins that includes antibodies, are produced in the liver, as are the proteins that make up the complement system, a part of the immune system that combines with antibodies to fight invading microorganisms.

Many other chemicals are produced by the liver. These include fibrinogen and prothrombin, which help wounds to heal by enabling blood to form clots, and cholesterol, a key component of cell membranes that transports fats in the bloodstream to body tissues.

In addition to manufacturing chemicals, the liver helps clear toxic substances, such as drugs and alcohol, from the bloodstream. It does this by absorbing the harmful substances, chemically altering them, and then excreting them in the bile.

Liver Diseases

Although the liver is exposed to many potentially harmful substances, it is a remarkable organ that is able to regenerate, or repair or replace, injured tissue. Its construction, in which many lobules perform the same task, means that if one section of the liver is damaged, another section will perform the functions of the injured area indefinitely or until the damaged section is repaired. But the liver is subject to many diseases that can overwhelm its regeneration abilities, threatening a person's health.

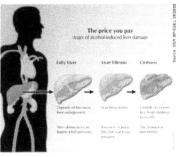

Diseases of the liver range from mild infection to life-threatening liver failure. For many of these ailments, the first sign of a problem is a condition called jaundice, characterized by a yellowish colouring of the skin and the whites of the eye. It develops when liver cells lose their ability to process bilirubin, the yellowish-brown pigment found in bile.

The liver can be harmed whenever injury or disease affects the rest of the body. For example, cancer may spread from the stomach or intestines to the liver, and diabetes, if not properly treated, may result in damage to the liver. Some diseases caused by parasites, including amebiasis and schistosomiasis, can damage the liver. Drug use, including long-term use of some prescription medications as well as illegal drugs, can also cause liver damage. Poisons can easily damage liver cells and even cause complete liver failure, especially the poisons found in certain mushrooms.

One of the most common liver diseases is hepatitis, an inflammation of the liver. Hepatitis may be caused by exposure to certain chemicals, by autoimmune diseases, or by bacterial infections. But hepatitis is most often caused by one of several viruses. The hepatitis A virus (HAV) can produce flulike symptoms and jaundice, but many people who contract it have no symptoms. The disease tends to resolve on its own. Because HAV lives in feces in the intestinal tract, hepatitis A is prevalent in areas where drinking water is contaminated with raw sewage. Good hygiene practices and a hepatitis A vaccination are effective measures of prevention.

Hepatitis B is a more serious ailment. Unlike HAV, hepatitis B virus (HBV) may remain active in the body for many years after the time of infection, sometimes permanently damaging the liver. HBV is found in blood and other body fluids—tears, saliva, and semen—and is spread through unprotected sexual intercourse and the sharing of infected needles or other sharp objects that puncture the skin.

In developed countries, alcohol-induced liver diseases far outnumber hepatitis and all other liver disorders. Heavy alcohol use causes fat deposits to build up in the liver, possibly leading to chronic hepatitis, which causes scarring and destruction of liver cells. Over many years, scarring in the liver can progress to cirrhosis, a disease characterized by diminished blood flow through this important organ. When this occurs, toxins are not adequately removed from the blood, blood pressure increases in the hepatic portal vein, and substances produced by the liver, such as blood proteins, are not adequately regulated. Cirrhosis cannot be reversed, but liver function can significantly improve in people who stop consuming alcohol during the early stages of this condition. Beyond abstinence from alcohol, treatments for cirrhosis may include drug therapy or surgery to redirect blood flow.

For people with severe liver disease or impending liver failure, organ transplantation may be an option. Unlike some organ transplants, such as kidney transplants, liver transplants are complex procedures that have not had high long-term success rates. Fortunately, new techniques and drugs are improving the outcome of liver transplants. Current success rates range between 60 and 80 percent, with more than half of recent transplant recipients surviving more than five years. Most of these people have an excellent prognosis for leading healthy, normal lives.

Beneficial Juices in Liver Ailments: Lemon, papaya, grapes, carrot, tomato, beet and cucumber.

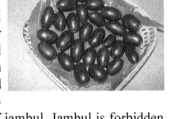

Jambul: In liver diseases, jambul-juice works like liver extract. Jambul should be soaked in cold water for an hour or two before juice is extracted. Jambul should not be taken on an empty stomach as it promotes windiness but can be had after meals. Milk should not be taken 3 hours before or after the consumption of jambul. Jambul is forbidden for a woman just after delivery or for one who observes fast. Jambul juice is many a time more effective than costly liver extract injections. Jambu is an excellent treatment for diabetes, indigestion, diarrhea, dysentery, kidney stones and leprosy and removes blood impurities.

Papaya : The ripe papaya increases virility, is beneficial to the heart, helps alleviate insanity, effective in liver troubles, is a good medicine for constipation, hyperacidity and urinary disorders, is helpful in expelling round worms from the digestive tract. In cases where patients 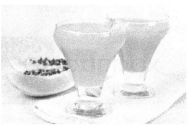 have taken a course of antibiotics, papaya is recommended to hasten the restoration of friendly symbiotic bacteria in the gut which would have been destroyed by drugs. Papaya cleanses the body completely. Papaya has been recommended for use as a part of treatment for cancer. It gives relief in asthma too. It is also known to help in menstrual disorders.

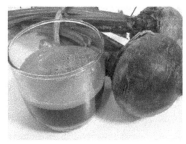 **Beetroot:** Beetroot juice is very powerful and should always be consumed in small quantities and usually mixed with other juices, such as apple, carrot, cucumber and celery. It is an excellent purifier and cleanser of the blood and is effective in cleaning out the liver, kidneys and arteries. Due to the high amounts of natural sugars that beetroot juice contains, it is thoroughly energising, although should be avoided by diabetics. It is also good for digestive problems such as constipation and it strengthens the bones, which is helpful for people as they get older and their bones become weaker.

Chapter 26
Neuritis

Neuritis is one of the serious nervous disorders, which refers to an inflammation of the nerves, involving a single nerve or a series of nerves. At times, several different groups of nerves in various parts of the body may be involved. This condition is known as polyneuritis; though this condition is not an inflammation, it is a change in the state of the nerves resulting in weakness, loss of the reflexes and changes of sensation.

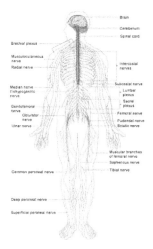

Symptoms of Neuritis

The main symptoms of neuritis are tingling, burning, and stabbing pains in the affected nerves. In severe cases, there may be numbness and loss of sensation and paralysis of the nearby muscles. Thus a temporary paralysis of the face may result from changes in the facial nerve on the affected side. During the acute stage of this condition, the patient may not be able to close the eyes due to loss of normal tone and strength by the muscles on the affected side of the face. Neuritis may also be caused by pernicious anemia, involving the nerves of the spine. The patient with this condition may find it very difficult to walk in the dark.

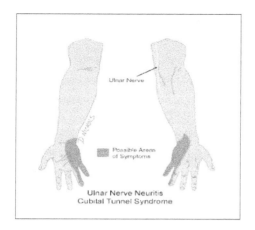

Ulnar Nerve

Possible Areas
of Symptoms

Ulnar Nerve Neuritis
Cubital Tunnel Syndrome

Causes of Neuritis

The chief cause of neuritis is chronic acidosis, that is, excessive acid condition of the blood and other body fluids. Wrong habits of living, overwork, etc., lower the tone of the nervous system and contribute towards neuritis. This disease can also result from a variety of nutritional deficiencies and metabolic disturbances such as faulty calcium metabolism, deficiencies of several B vitamins like B12, B6, B1, pantothenic acid and B2 and general toxaemia.

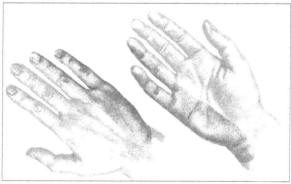

Other causes of neuritis include a blow, a penetrating injury, a bad bruise or heavy pressure over a nerve trunk and dislocation and fractures of the bones. Any violent muscular activity or over-extension of the joint as in sprains may injure the nerves and cause neuritis. The condition may also result from certain infections such as tuberculosis, diptheria, tetanus, leprosy and diabetes mellitus, poisoning with insecticides, mercury, lead, arsenic and alcohol.

Treatment of Neuritis by Nature Cure
Diet:
The best treatment for neuritis is to ensure that the patient gets optimum nutrition, well assimilated with all the vitamins and other nutrients. The emphasis should be on whole grains, particularly whole wheat, brown rice, raw and sprouted seeds, raw milk, especially in soured form, and home made cottage cheese. In this regimen, the breakfast may consist of fresh fruits, a handful of raw nuts or a couple of tablespoons of sunflower and pumpkin seeds. Steamed vegetables, whole-wheat chappatis and a glass of buttermilk may be taken for lunch. The dinner may comprise a large bowl of fresh, green, vegetable salad, fresh home-made cottage cheese, fresh butter and a glass of butter-milk.

All vitamins of the B group have proved highly beneficial in the prevention and treatment of neuritis. The disorder has been helped when vitamins B1, B2, B6, B12 and pantothenic acid have been given together, and extreme pain weakness and numbness in some cases have been relieved within an hour. In severe cases, the patient should be put on a short juice fast for four or five days before being given the optimum diet. Carrot, beet, citrus fruits, apple and pineapple may be used for juices. The patient should avoid white bread, white sugar, refined cereals, meat, fish, tinned foods, tea, coffee and condiments which are at the root of the trouble, by continuously flooding the tissues with acid impurities.

Home Remedies
Certain remedies have been found highly beneficial in the treatment of neuritis. One such remedy is soybean milk. Soyabean milk is prepared by soaking the beans in water for about 12 hours. The skin of the beans is then removed and after a thorough wash, they are turned into a fine paste in a grinding machine. The paste is mixed with water three times its quantity. The milk should then be boiled on slow fire, stirring it frequently. After it becomes little cooler, it should be strained through a cheesecloth and sugar added. This cupful of soybean milk mixed with a teaspoonful of honey should be taken every night in this condition. It tones up the nervous system due to its rich concentration of lecithin, vitamin B and glutanic acid.

Barley brew is another effective remedy for neuritis. It is prepared by boiling one-quarter cup of all natural pearled barley in two quarters of water. When the water has boiled down to about one quarter, it should be strained carefully. For better results, it should be mixed with buttermilk and limejuice. Raw carrot and spinach have proved valuable in neuritis, as both these vegetables are rich in elements. The quickest and most effective way in which the body can obtain and assimilate these elements is by drinking daily at least half a litre of the combined raw juices of carrot and spinach.

Beneficial Juices in Neuritis: Orange, pineapple, apple, carrot and beet.

Carrot and Spinach Juice
Some people do not know the benefits of carrot juice just yet. Carrot juice has proven to be beneficial in more ways than one and curing neuritis is one of them. Make a mixed vegetable juice of carrot and spinach juice by combining three-fifths of a glass of carrot juice with two-fifths of a glass of spinach juice. Consume this combination daily.

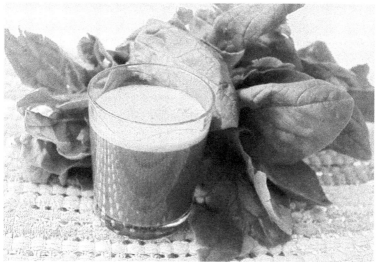

Celery Juice and Neuritis
Neuritis, also called neuropathy, is the term used for damage to your nerves. It may be caused by an injury or by a systemwide ailment,

such as diabetes or high blood pressure. Neuritis may cause a tingling or burning sensation, loss of sensation, weakness, paralysis or a combination of these symptoms. Celery juice is included in some alternative medicine remedies for this condition. Talk to your doctor for a proper diagnosis and treatment plan before trying any remedy for neuritis.

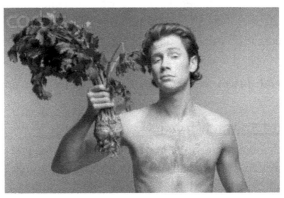

Significance
You must identify the cause of your neuritis to treat it properly. For example, if it's caused by diabetes or high blood pressure you need to treat the underlying problem. Your doctor may recommend corticosteroids or surgery if your neuritis is caused by an entrapped nerve. She also might prescribe pain medication or antidepressants. Sometimes no treatment is needed and your neuritis will resolve on its own. Celery juice is used in traditional medicine remedies for two underlying causes of neuritis -- high blood pressure and diabetes.

Celery Juice and High Blood Pressure
Celery has a theoretical benefit if your neuritis is caused by high blood pressure because it contains substances such as the plant chemicals 3-n-butyl phthalide and apigenin that help lower blood pressure. Apigenin is a vasodilator, meaning it dilates your blood vessels. However, the 3-n-butyl phthalide is believed to be celery's key blood-pressure lowering ingredient. In addition to dilating your blood vessels it reduces levels of stress hormones in your blood, according to the Reader's Digest publication, "Eat to Beat Blood Pressure," by Robyn Webb and Jamy D. Ard. Juicing four stalks of

celery supplies a therapeutic dose of these plant chemicals. Consult a doctor before using this traditional medicine remedy and have medical supervision if you do use celery to as a hypertension therapy because more research is needed to determine whether celery juice is effective for this use.

The Diabetes Connection

Neuropathy, or neuritis, is a common complication in diabetes. Celery also is used in traditional Chinese medicine in diet therapy for treating diabetes. Diabetes is characterized in TCM as a condition that has, in part, excess internal heat. Celery is on the list of TCM foods that have a cooling effect on the body, according to an August 2001 scientific review published in "Diabetes Spectrum." If you use TCM to treat diabetes, be sure to do so under the supervision of a health care professional who monitors your blood glucose levels, recommends review author Maggie B. Covington. That's because, while TCM may help optimize your body's ability to function normally, it does not offer a cure for diabetes and more research on effectiveness and safety of TCM diabetes remedies is needed, Covington notes.

Use

Celery juice is often paired other juices in alternative medicine treatments for neuritis. For example, celery, carrot and parsley juice is one recommended combination, according to "Alternative Medicine," by Larry Trivieri and John W. Anderson. While you can use this treatment at home, you need to do so under the supervision of a qualified alternative medicine professional because the juice therapy is likely to be just one component of your therapy, the authors note. For example, the practitioner might also recommend dietary changes such as increasing your fluid intake, consuming whole foods instead of processed foods, and avoiding stimulating foods like caffeine and refined sugar.

Considerations

Celery juice does not commonly cause side effects, though it can have a diuretic effect. However celery can interact with certain medications. Taking it with certain antibiotics such as doxycycline and some anti-inflammatory medications like ibuprofen can increase your skin's sensitivity to sunlight. Using celery with fondaparinux can raise your risk for bleeding and bruising. Using it with leothyroxine can reduce effectiveness of this drug. Celery also is contraindicated if you have a kidney ailment because it may trigger inflammation.